AF737234

'If Bion and Winnicott were to have had a discussion, what might it have been like? The need for this conversation to happen has passed down through the analytic generations and has here reached a very challenging and informed expression in the hands of Abram and Hinshelwood'.

Nicola Abel-Hirsch, *training and supervising analyst BPaS and author of* Bion: 365 Quotes

'This second book in the series authored by Jan Abram and Bob Hinshelwood fulfils its promise of opening up discussion and debate about the work of Wilfred Bion and Donald W. Winnicott. These two giants of mid-twentieth century psychoanalysis were both born before the turn of the century but were of different psychoanalytic generations. They were both personally marked by the horrors of the world wars, which in different ways affected their contributions to psychoanalysis, as they each took the influence of Melanie Klein in radically different directions. There is a freshness and immediacy to the to-and-fro of the dialogue between these two experts in their field, which follows the exposition of Bion and Winnicott's central concepts. The dialogue does much to shed light on the often confused equivalences that have been made between such concepts as "holding" in Winnicott and "container-contained" in Bion, both emphasising the differing roots in each conceptual frame and their consequence for clinical practice. The exchanges between Abram and Hinshelwood are exploratory and frank, respectful and challenging. In our discipline, which can sometimes divide along partisan lines, this is a refreshing and informative read'.

Angela Joyce, *training and supervising analyst BPaS, former chair The Winnicott Trust*

'Jan Abram and R.D. Hinshelwood are famous for their scholarship on the Winnicott and Kleinian tradition respectively, integrated in a great clinical experience. In this book they compare Winnicott and Bion head-to-head qua background, evolution, major concepts and psychoanalytic practice. The result is refreshing and easy to read. Not only the differences but also the common background (for example, Klein's influence) and the intertwinement of their concepts are highlighted. I enjoyed the lively discussion between Abram and Hinshelwood at the end of each part, which often led to surprising new points of view'.

Rudi Vermote, *training and supervising analyst, Belgian Psychoanalytic Society, author of* Reading Bion

The Clinical Paradigms of DONALD WINNICOTT and WILFRED BION

This book introduces the psychoanalytic principles of both Winnicott and Bion, to compare the ways in which their concepts evolved, and to show how their different approaches contribute to distinctive psychoanalytic paradigms that warrant further research.

The book is comprised of five parts, each of which ends with a dialogue between the authors, to provide an in-depth look at the perspectives of Winnicott and Bion on the following issues: the British Psychoanalytical Society; working with children and groups; the formulation of psychoanalytic principles; the consolidation of their ideas and new beginnings; and their clinical approaches. Structuring an analysis of Winnicott and Bion's work in this way simultaneously acts as a comprehensive introduction to their thinking and provokes further research into the ways in which the Winnicottian and Bionian traditions interact.

The Clinical Paradigms of Donald Winnicott and Wilfred Bion will appeal to all those seeking an introduction to psychoanalytic ideas and to these two schools of British Object Relations especially.

Jan Abram is a training and supervising psychoanalyst of the British Psychoanalytical Society and visiting professor of the Psychoanalysis Unit, University College, London. She is vice-president of the European Psychoanalytic Federation. She has published several books and articles notably: *The Language of Winnicott* (1st edition 1996; 2nd edition 2007), which was judged Outstanding Academic Book of the Year (1997); *Donald Winnicott Today* (2013); *The Surviving Object: Psychoanalytic Clinical Essays on Psychic Survival-of-the-Object* (2022).

R.D. Hinshelwood is a fellow of the British Psychoanalytical Society and of the Royal College of Psychiatrists. He has written widely on clinical psychoanalysis and its wider applications to society, politics and ethics as well as comparative research methods.

ROUTLEDGE CLINICAL PARADIGMS DIALOGUE SERIES

Jan Abram and R.D. Hinshelwood
Series Editors

Under the joint editorship of Jan Abram and R.D. Hinshelwood, the *Routledge Clinical Paradigms Dialogue* book series will develop studies of conceptual research by promoting dialogue between different psychoanalytic theories. Following the success of their co-authored book, *The Clinical Paradigms of Melanie Klein and Donald Winnicott: Comparisons and Dialogues*, which introduced the distinctive psychoanalytic principles of both Klein and Winnicott together, the editors proposed this series in order to show, through the unique format of a dialogue, how the distinct schools of psychoanalytic thought have evolved and how certain misunderstandings have arisen.

Books in the series follow the same format as the original book, with each being written about two prominent psychoanalytic authors by two internationally recognised scholars. Through these unique pairings, each book will engage in systematic, extended examinations of the similarities and differences between psychoanalytic orientations, setting them apart from existing literature in psychoanalysis.

The volumes in this series will appeal to clinical practitioners in practice and in training who have different levels of knowledge and experience of psychoanalysis, and to any with an interest in comparing and dialoguing between the psychoanalytic schools of thought.

For more information about this series, please visit: www.routledge.com/Routledge-Clinical-Paradigms-Dialogue-Series/book-series/RCPD

The Clinical Paradigms of Melanie Klein and Donald Winnicott
Comparisons and Dialogues
Jan Abram and R.D. Hinshelwood

The Clinical Paradigms of Donald Winnicott and Wilfred Bion
Comparisons and Dialogues
Jan Abram and R.D. Hinshelwood

The Clinical Paradigms of DONALD WINNICOTT and WILFRED BION

Comparisons and Dialogues

Jan Abram and R.D. Hinshelwood

Routledge
Taylor & Francis Group
LONDON AND NEW YORK

Designed cover image: Wilfred R. Bion (right), photographed by Michael Paul and here reprinted courtesy of the Estate of W.R. Bion, and Donald Winnicott (left).

First published 2023
by Routledge
4 Park Square, Milton Park, Abingdon, Oxon OX14 4RN

and by Routledge
605 Third Avenue, New York, NY 10158

Routledge is an imprint of the Taylor & Francis Group, an informa business

© 2023 Jan Abram and R.D. Hinshelwood

The right of Jan Abram and R.D. Hinshelwood to be identified as authors of this work has been asserted in accordance with sections 77 and 78 of the Copyright, Designs and Patents Act 1988.

All rights reserved. No part of this book may be reprinted or reproduced or utilised in any form or by any electronic, mechanical, or other means, now known or hereafter invented, including photocopying and recording, or in any information storage or retrieval system, without permission in writing from the publishers.

Trademark notice: Product or corporate names may be trademarks or registered trademarks, and are used only for identification and explanation without intent to infringe.

British Library Cataloguing-in-Publication Data
A catalogue record for this book is available from the British Library

Every effort has been made to contact copyright holders. Please advise the publisher of any errors or omissions, and these will be corrected in subsequent editions.

ISBN: 9781032465807 (hbk)
ISBN: 9781032465821 (pbk)
ISBN: 9781003382409 (ebk)

DOI: 10.4324/9781003382409

Typeset in Palatino
by Newgen Publishing UK

To those who have taught us and to those we have taught
and
For all those who have engaged in this project
On comparisons and dialogues, at home and abroad.

CONTENTS

ACKNOWLEDGEMENTS

Our acknowledgments in the first book of this series, *The Clinical Paradigms of Melanie Klein and Donald Winnicott: Comparisons and Dialogues*, still stand. The reception of that book encouraged us to start this book, and we are pleased that Routledge has commissioned a series following the same format we have now used for both books. We wish to acknowledge all those colleagues who have continued to offer us feedback on the need for comparisons and dialogues, and while we have shown that it has its challenges, we hope we have also demonstrated how possible it is to make an effort at least to dialogue with each other. Jan and Bob acknowledge each other for not only continuing to retain the interest in completing this book but also for Bob's considerable patience in Jan's finding the time to get on with this project, finally! And for Jan for leading with so much energy and competence.

Not least, we would like to thank our forgiving spouses and family, who tolerated our obsessive emailing during certain intensive stages of the dialogues.

Jan Abram (Vale of Glamorgan, Summer 2022)
R.D. Hinshelwood (Norfolk, Summer 2022)

ABOUT THE AUTHORS

R.D. Hinshelwood trained in medicine at University College Hospital in London, graduating with both a BSc (in anatomy) as well as an MBBS. His training as a psychiatrist took him to Shenley Hospital (1967–1969), where he published his first papers (one in *Nature*, and one in the *British Journal of Psychiatry*), and then to the Marlborough Day Hospital (1969–1976) and the experience of developing a co-operative-style therapeutic community with colleagues there. During that time he gained his diploma in Psychological Medicine; he also entered his own personal analysis, with a view to training as a psychoanalyst with the British Psychoanalytical Society, where he qualified in 1976.

He was then appointed consultant psychotherapist to St Bernard's Hospital in 1976, where he developed psychoanalytically informed courses and support for mental health staff. This has become a life-long interest in the psychodynamics of psychiatric and other organisations and the practical consequences of this stressful work; he wrote a number of publications in this area including *Observing Organisations* (Hinshelwood and Skogstad, 2001). During the 1970s and the 1980s, he was active in the developing world of psychoanalytic psychotherapy, teaching on the training course of a number of organisations, in the course of which he mastered the intricacies of Melanie Klein's thought and wrote *A Dictionary of Kleinian Thought* (1989; 2nd edition 1991), now translated into a dozen languages. In 1984 he founded the *British Journal of Psychotherapy*, editing it for ten years, and in 1996 he founded *Psychoanalysis and History*, publishing both journals until 2006. He became a member of the Royal College of Psychiatrists in 1990 and a fellow in 1993. One outcome of this period was his book *Suffering Insanity* (2004).

In 1993, he moved from his consultant role at St Bernard's (which had become Ealing Hospital) to become director of the Cassel Hospital (the longstanding therapeutic community founded by Tom Main). He retired from the NHS in 1997 and was then appointed as professor at the Centre for Psychoanalytic Studies at the University of Essex. In 2002 he was visiting professor at the Committee on Social Thought, University of Chicago. The academic world offered an opportunity to consider the study of clinical psychoanalysis and the problem of comparative studies between rival psychoanalytic schools; this led to "Repression and Splitting: Towards a Method of Conceptual Comparison" (2008) and *Research on the Couch: Single Case Studies, Subjectivity and Psychoanalytic Knowledge* (2003). In 2016 he published *Countertransference and Alive Moments*. His interests include, of course, the events and publications connected with this present book with Jan Abram.

Jan Abram is a training and supervising psychoanalyst of the British Psychoanalytical Society, in private practice in London. She is visiting professor of the Psychoanalysis Unit, University College, London, where she teaches and has convened courses for the MSc in Psychoanalytic Studies. She is a visiting lecturer in the Adult Department, Tavistock Clinic, London. Since 2008 she was a member of the Paris Group, a research group of the European Psychoanalytical Federation (EPF) and a working party of the International Psychoanalytic Association for "the Specificity of Psychoanalytic Treatment Today". She was chair of the group between 2016 and 2019. Between 2011 and 2013 she was visiting professor for the Centre for Psychoanalytic Studies, University of Essex. Later in 2016 she was visiting professor at Kyoto University, Kyoto, Japan, on a three-month writing sabbatical. During this time she lectured, taught and supervised and co-authored with R.D. Hinshelwood *The Clinical Paradigms of Melanie Klein and Donald Winnicott: Comparisons and Dialogues* (2018). During this sabbatical she also prepared the synopsis for her collection of clinical papers *The Surviving Object: psychoanalytic clinical essays on psychic survival of the object*, which was published by the New Library of Psychoanalysis, Routledge, in 2022.

Abram lectures, teaches and supervises at home and abroad. She is vice president for the EPF for the Annual Conferences and was formerly chair of the Scientific Committee (BPaS).

Jan Abram has published several books and articles notably: *The Language of Winnicott* (1st edition 1996; 2nd edition 2007), which received Outstanding Academic Book of the year in 1997; *Donald Winnicott Today* (2013) – shortlisted for the Gradiva Award for Edited volumes; *The Clinical Paradigms of Melanie Klein and Donald Winnicott: Comparisons and Dialogues* (2018, with co-author R.D. Hinshelwood); and most recently a collection of her clinical essays, *The Surviving Object: psychoanalytic clinical essays on psychic survival of the object*, published by New Library of Psychoanalysis, Routledge. With R.D. Hinshelwood she is series editor for the Routledge Clinical Paradigms Dialogues Series.

For more details on both authors go to:

janabram.com

www.psychoanalysis.org.uk/our-authors-and-theorists/jan-abram-0

www.rdhinshelwood.net

PREFACE

As we have already stated in our first book of this series, this book arose out of our work at the University of Essex in 2011. Both of us have enjoyed the challenge of attempting to have a neutral dialogue with each other from our different theoretical paradigms: R.D. Hinshelwood from Klein and Bion's, and Jan Abram from Winnicott's clinical paradigm. The first book in the series, *The Clinical Paradigms of Melanie Klein and Donald Winnicott*, has been received with much interest from experienced analysts as well as beginners in psychoanalysis. This has been encouraging enough for us to continue with the project and to publish a book, following the same format, on comparing perhaps two of the most currently well-known authors, Donald Winnicott and Wilfred Bion.

Our main aim with the structure of the books is to retain a sense of the lively and spontaneous interchanges we had achieved in the workshops and conferences we gave. To that end, the book steps out of the mould of psychoanalytic publications, as it is an attempt to create a dialogue between two major thinkers in psychoanalysis after Freud, Ferenczi, and Lacan.

If we look back to Plato, we are reminded that the aims of the Socratic method were to facilitate a "cooperative argumentative between individuals based on questioning and answering questions in order to stimulate critical thinking and to draw out ideas and underlying presumptions". Following these aims, we found that there was a considerable need to make some differences between psychoanalytical paradigms much clearer, as the adherents of each framework of ideas had not only a deficient understanding of the other but also active misunderstanding in some respects.

This book, like the first in the series, is divided into five parts. Since Winnicott was the prior analyst, it made sense that Jan Abram started each part. Thus the core of this book is made up of ten chapters and five dialogues.

The dialogues are made up of a series of emails between the authors, and it was important to retain a sense of flow, which meant that most of the dialogues, at least, occurred during several breaks during the analytic year: September to August 2019–2022. The manuscript for this book was compiled during the summer of 2022.

We both feel that, like the first book, we have learnt a tremendous amount. Our overall aim has been to make the book both short and accessible. This inevitably means that there are limitations to the scope of the book, as our effort has been to home in on the main convergences and divergences between our protagonists – Donald Winnicott and Wilfred Bion.

As we said in our first book, we hope again that the road we have taken together can be freshly and fruitfully trodden by all readers, so as to provide insight into the rich details and nuances that can be discovered through this compare-and-contrast approach.

CHRONOLOGIES

Donald Winnicott (1896–1971)	Wilfred Bion (1897–1979)
Born 1896 Plymouth, Devon 1910 Boarding school, The Leys School, Cambridge 1914 Pre-medical course, Jesus College Cambridge 1917 Surgeon probationer, Royal Navy 1919 Reads Freud's Interpretation of Dreams 1920–1922 Qualifies in medicine – specialises in paediatrics 1923 Two hospital appointments Queen's Hospital for Children, Hackney, and Consultant Paddington Green Children's Hospital 1923 Begins analysis with James Strachey 1924 Sets up in private practice 1927 Registers as a candidate at the Institute of Psychoanalysis 1929 Begins to attend Scientific Meetings of the British Psychoanalytical Society (BPaS)	Born 1897 in Mathura (Northern India) 1905 Sent to Bishop Stortford School, and never returned to India 1915 Conscripted into the army 1917–1918 Commander of a tank battalion 1919–1921 Attends Queens College, Oxford, studying history and philosophy. Teaches at Bishops Stortford School 1922–1923 Travels in France Late 1920s and early 1930s Medical training at University College Hospital Medical School After registration as a doctor, Bion briefly holds a part-time appointment at the Queens Square Hospital for Nervous Diseases and at a private medical practice 1934 Begins psychotherapy training at the Tavistock Clinic. He has some psychotherapy with J.A. Hadfield 1935 Appointed to the staff of the Tavistock Clinic

1931 First publication, "Clinical Notes on Disorders of Childhood" 1933 Terminates analysis with James Strachey 1934 Qualifies as a psychoanalyst for adults 1935 Qualifies as the first male child analyst 1935 Becomes a full member of the British Psychoanalytical Society. Reading-in paper: "The manic defence" (1958) 1935–41 Consultations with Melanie Klein and second analysis with Joan Riviere 1941 Named by Melanie Klein as one of the five Kleinian analysts 1941 "Dropped" by Klein Phase Two: Transitional phenomena (1945–1960) 1945 Presents "Primitive emotional development" to the British Psychoanalytical Society 1947 Presents "Hate in the countertransference" to the BpaS 1948 Presents "Reparation in respect of mother's organised defence against depression" 1951 Presents "Transitional objects and transitional phenomena" to the BPaS 1954 Presents "Metapsychological and clinical aspects of regression within the psychoanalytical set-up" to the BpaS 1956 Becomes president of the BPaS 1957 Two new publications: "The child and the family: first relationships" and "The child and the outside world: studies in developing relationships". Presents "The capacity to be alone" to the BPaS 1958 Publication of Collected Papers: Through Paediatrics To Psychoanalysis Phase Three: The use of an object (1960–1971) 1960 Presents "The theory of the	Group Period 1938 Starts an analysis with John Rickman, which lasts only 18 months because of the commencement of the war in 1939 1941 Marries the actress Betty Jardine. Joins the EMS (Emergency Medical Service) 1942 Joins Army Psychiatric Service and the team developing the War Office Selection Boards (WOSB) to recruit officers from the ranks after Dunkirk. Late 1942 Moves to Northfield Hospital and is placed in charge of the rehabilitation wing January 1943 Conducts the Northfield experiment using social field theory for six weeks. Publishes in the Lancet a joint paper with John Rickman about the Northfield experiment 1943 Returns to setting up more WOSB teams 1945 His wife dies three days after giving birth to their first child, Parthenope. He begins both an analysis with Klein and his training at the Institute of Psychoanalysis in London 1946 He commences his first training patient under supervision with Paula Heimann 1948 Publishes a paper. "Group methods of treatment", wherein he prioritises countertransference over transference. Psychosis research 1950 Becomes a member of the British Psychoanalytical Society (BPaS) and joins a research group developing Klein's theory of schizoid mechanisms (with Hanna Segal and Herbert Rosenfeld) 1953 His first paper on schizophrenia is presented to the International Psychoanalytical Association at the Edinburgh Congress, published 1954

parent-infant relationship" and writes "Ego distortion in terms of true and false self" 1962 Presents "The development of the capacity for concern" and "Morals and education" to the BPaS 1963 Retires from Paddington Green. Presents "Communicating and not communicating leading to a study of certain opposites" 1964 Publishes The Child, the Family and the Outside World with Penguin Books 1965 Becomes president of the BpaS for the second time. Publishes "The family and individual development" and prepares an introduction for a book on sixteen sessions with a small child which will be published posthumously in 1977 – The Piggle (1967). Publishes "Mirror-role of mother and family in child development" 1968 Awarded the James Spence Medal for Paediatrics and presents "The use of an object" to the New York Psychoanalytical Society. 1969 Writes on and around "The use of an object" and prepares to publish two books: Playing and Reality and Therapeutic Consultations (which will be published later in 1971) 1970 Writes on the themes of creativity 1971 Prepares a paper for the 27th International Psychoanalytical Association congress to be held in Vienna on "The psychoanalytical concept of aggression: theoretical, clinical and applied aspects". Dies on January 25th	1959 Delivers his seminal paper on container-contained, inferring a communicative form of projective identification 1960 Melanie Klein dies. Bion becomes chair of the Melanie Klein Trust Epistemology of psychoanalysis 1962 Bion begins a series of publications on the epistemology of psychoanalysis, in effect a Kleinian metapsychology – *Learning from Experience* (1962), *Elements of Psychoanalysis* (1963), *Transformations* (1965) 1962–1965 Becomes president of the BPaS 1967 Bion publishes a book of his papers on psychotic states, and in an extended commentary repudiates the earlier work as impossible for anyone to understand who could not be present in the sessions from which the material was quoted. He never after published clinical material. 1968 After a successful lecture and seminar tour in Los Angeles, Bion moved there with the encouragement of Albert Masson. 1969– Bion travels to a number of countries to give clinical seminars and lectures which he never publishes in his lifetime. Intuition and the aesthetics of psychoanalysis 1970 Publishes his book *Attention and Interpretation*, exploring his uncertainty about what sort of discipline psychoanalysis is, and promoting the importance of intuition over symbolic and verbal communication.

	1975–1979 Publishes three novels as if he were considering the importance of an aesthetic approach (or vertex) as opposed to the scientific approach to psychoanalysis. 1979 Bion returns to England, plans a visit to India for the first time since childhood, but dies within three months of his return on 8 November.

Introduction

This book follows the structure of the first book in the series – *The Clinical Paradigms of Melanie Klein and Donald Winnicott* – which aimed firstly to compare two different psychoanalytic paradigms and secondly to dialogue about their differences. As with the first book, there are five parts, each with two chapters on the general theme and a more systematic brief summary of the main concepts that emerge. This is followed in each part by a dialogue, initiated by Abram, in response to both authors' reading of each other's chapter. The dialogues were conducted by email. We tried to retain the spontaneous nature of the dialogues. In fact, following the first book we published, very little of our email exchanges have been edited and the reader will notice emerging tensions from time to time which we felt were important to retain in order to convey the kind of difficulties that inevitably occur when a dialogue on differences is attempted. Our aim has been to highlight differences and to try to avoid competition about our two authors, despite both of us having a clear favourite.

This short introduction signals the themes and discussions that grew spontaneously out of the chapters and throughout the course of each dialogue.

Part I sets out a general overview of Donald Winnicott and Wilfred Bion in the context of the British Psychoanalytical Society in which they

DOI: 10.4324/9781003382409-1

evolved their theories. While they were born only a year apart, Donald Winnicott qualified as a psychoanalyst in 1934, while Wilfred Bion, despite his important work hitherto, qualified in 1950 (see "Chronologies").

What becomes very clear in the chapters is that both men were significantly traumatised by their experience during WW1: Winnicott in the navy as a medic on a destroyer and Bion in the army mostly on active service as commander of a company of tanks. In Chapter 1, Abram presents Winnicott's biographical background, showing how he came to discover psychoanalysis after returning from the experience of being a surgeon probationer in the final months of WW1. Parallel with that experience, Hinshelwood's Chapter 2 presents Bion's account of one of his colleagues dying in his arms. Implicit in both chapters is the question of why both men chose psychoanalysis as a therapeutic method. Later in their work, their trauma does perhaps become a significant theme in their formulations of individual emotional development, as we shall see.

In Chapter 1 – "Donald Winnicott and the Kleinian development" – Abram shows how Winnicott's early study to become a psychoanalyst and child analyst was very much influenced by the pioneering work of Melanie Klein, who had settled in London since 1926 after coming from Berlin via Budapest. From his ten-year analysis with James Strachey, who had been analysed by Sigmund Freud himself, Winnicott's main influence was classical Freudian analysis. But as a paediatrician, Winnicott's perspective on the infantile in each distressed adult – including himself – inevitably meant he was acutely aware of the infant's point of view. The latter perspective was facilitated through regression in the psychoanalytic clinical setting, which, for Winnicott, became the means of appreciating infantile states of mind. This became his abiding experience and belief through the ineffable experience of the Freudian psychoanalytic method.

Chapter 2 – "Wilfred Bion and Klein's schizoid mechanisms" – starts with an evocation of Bion's account of a fellow soldier gasping his last words at the moment of death from an appalling injury. Bion wrote that he never recovered from this event, saying he had also died on that day. Later, some therapy and his work at the Tavistock Centre in London in its early days meant that Bion came into contact with psychoanalysis. Bion came to train as an analyst when he was already a "celebrated authority" on group therapy, and his training analyst during his training as a psychoanalyst was Melanie Klein. As his training took place in the aftermath of the Controversial Discussions period, this meant that he followed a Kleinian training and was thus designated a follower of Klein from the beginning of his entrance into the institute. Hinshelwood's thesis in this chapter is that what interested Bion most of all in Klein's work was her work on the paranoid-schizoid position. Unlike Winnicott, Bion did not become a child analyst and had no real experience of paediatrics. However, he had three babies of his own; for the first of whom he became the sole parent after the death of his wife immediately after childbirth.

The Part I dialogue, initiated by Abram after reading Hinshelwood's Chapter 2, starts with a perhaps maternal concern about Bion's early childhood when, at the age of eight, he was sent from his parental home in India to a boarding school in the UK. Winnicott was also sent to boarding school, but not till he was 14, and only a matter of 300 miles away – from Plymouth to Cambridge. Survivor guilt, as a consequence of the many deaths of close colleagues they witnessed in combat, is a factor for both men, and in the dialogue this cannot be ignored. But Abram shows interest in Bion's mother: Where was she in Hinshelwood's narrative?

Hinshelwood agrees with the probability that both men suffered survivor guilt, and his answer to the question about Bion's mother is that as a child, Bion was very attached to his Ayah. This, Hinshelwood believes, is why Bion showed an interest in mysticism in his late work.

What emerges in the dialogue is that Winnicott formulated a theory of trauma which evolved from his work in paediatrics alongside his personal analysis. He was convinced that the baby will be traumatised or not due to the deficiency of the environment from birth onwards. Hinshelwood makes clear that for Kleinians, infantile anxiety constitutes the paranoid-schizoid position, which is universal and occurs to every baby at the very start of life. Abram's response is that for Winnicott and those following his paradigm the paranoid-schizoid position depicts a "deficiency" of the holding environment rather than being a universal, inner psychic state.

Abram and Hinshelwood agree on the connection between intrapsychic and interpsychic dynamics from the beginning of life in both Winnicott's and Bion's work, but it is striking that the dialogue also brings out both men's early experience of their mothers. Many questions are implicitly raised which are not answered in relation to family dynamics. Winnicott comes out as more emotionally privileged than Bion due to his large family surrounding him as he was growing up. Winnicott's epiphany that "there's no such thing as a baby" in 1942 arrived before Bion started his training.

This first dialogue revisits some of the themes of the first book that relate to major differences between the Kleinian theoretical development and Winnicott's divergence from certain concepts. This defines the fundamental conflictual areas that inevitably arise between Winnicott and Bion, because despite the innovations that Bion clearly brought to the development of psychoanalysis, it is clear that his fundamental clinical paradigm is that of Klein. The next chapters and dialogue tease out how Bion advanced the Kleinian paradigm.

In Part II – "Analytic work with children and groups" – Chapters 3 and 4 introduce the very different professions of each man. Winnicott chose medicine and specialised in paediatrics, while Bion studied history and philosophy. In Chapter 3 – "Babies and their families" – Abram outlines the historical evolution of Winnicott's formulations, indicating that his clinical paradigm could be seen to amount to a "Kuhnian scientific revolution". The "environment-individual setup" or the claim that "there's no such thing as a baby" is Winnicott's starting point in revolutionising the Freudian paradigm. For Freud, psychosexuality shaped the individual's psyche, but for Winnicott the "fact of dependency" preceded psychosexuality in human development. Transitional phenomena and the use of an object were major formulations in Winnicott's thought that emerged out of the parental holding that structured mental growth.

In Chapter 4 – "Psychodynamics and the psychosocial" – Hinshelwood shows how Bion's trajectory towards psychoanalysis was via group dynamics. Early on he was very influenced by the way in which he observed his early mentor, Wilfred Trotter, listening to patients. Later in his training at the institute, Trotter's approach tied in with Klein's approach, who also advocated "learning from the patient" through attentive listening to the patient's perspective.

In the dialogue, Abram is struck by how Bion's emphasis on listening to the patient as the "fount of all knowledge" is in line with Winnicott's approach. The question of how this is conveyed to the patient develops into a line of inquiry about technique in the analytic encounter. How does the analyst deal with the patient's intolerable affects? These themes relate to the early controversies between Anna Freud's way of working and Melanie Klein's. The dialogue refers back to the history of psychoanalysis and its conflicts as well as forwards to the distinctions between a Winnicott-framed technique and a Bion-framed technique. There are many points of agreement in relation to listening to the patient, but in terms of technique there are differences that start to be articulated in relation to the central concepts of both authors; that is, holding, for Winnicott, and container-contained, for Bion. This dialogue concludes with more differentiation, which leads into Part III of the book – "The principle formulations".

Holding and containing are, by now, very well-known concepts in the psychoanalytic literature. Chapters 5 and 6 aim to outline the meaning of these celebrated theories. Are they the same concepts with different clothes? Or do they appear to be more similar than they actually are?

In Chapter 5 – "Holding" – Abram offers a brief history of the nature of holding and relates how clear it is in Winnicott's work that it basically depicts the crucial fact of the mother's psyche and how her maternal dedication to her infant is absolutely key to the infant's mental health. Winnicott was evolving this theory from the 1940s and continued to elaborate the concepts until his very late work.

In Chapter 6 – "Transformations" – Hinshelwood outlines Bion's formulations on the container-contained and describes how it became a paradigm for clinical technique. Contrary to Winnicott, Bion, following Klein, did not see containing as ameliorating the infant's anxiety about the survival of its sense of self. The mother's containing came about through her "reverie", which meant she could make meaning of the infant's intolerable feelings, like the feeling of dying, and thus enable the infant to make sense for himself (and increase the ego functions and the self).

In the dialogue, Abram wishes to clarify the differences between the concepts and shows her concern that Hinshelwood, like many others, has misunderstood Winnicott's concept of holding as being less complex than the container-contained. Both Abram and Hinshelwood are interested in Strachey's concept of the "therapeutic action" of psychoanalysis, and as they exchange their different authors' perspectives and introduce the distinct terms and phrases used by both Winnicott and Bion, further elaboration and distinctions are attempted. At times, the dialogue veers into a more philosophical position – Hinshelwood wonders if Winnicott was more of a positivist than Bion; later discussion turns to Abram's recent experience of teaching the MSc at University College London and her experience of clinical practice between schools of psychoanalysis in the British Psychoanalytical Society today. Finally, they agree to move on to Part IV, although Hinshelwood continues to be concerned that the real meanings of interpretation and technique have not yet been defined – at least not by Abram.

Chapters 7 and 8 in Part IV – "Consolidation and new beginnings" – continue to elaborate on the resonances between the authors and show how they share many overlapping concerns and themes. But it is quite noticeable that these points of convergence are not acknowledged by either author.

In Chapter 7 – "From primary maternal preoccupation to the use of an object" – Abram focuses on the late concepts of Winnicott that emerged from his early work on the maternal. Increasingly, she notes,

Winnicott laid greater stress on the mother's psychic contribution to the nascent psyche. The father will have no chance if the mother does not allow him in by introducing the infant to the father. This is why the mother is all powerful. There is a sequence of five stages in early object-relating for Winnicott that Abram dissects and defines as the "new feature" introduced in 1968.

In Chapter 8 – "Rethinking and making an impact" – Hinshelwood shows a more erratic progress in the work of Bion, who became increasingly interested in the nature of listening and how the patient deals with pre-conceptions. Strongly influenced by his student years spent studying philosophy, Bion picked up on Kantian notions as he formulated a specific language to signify aspects of the psyche. The "invariant" and "intuition" became key to his late formulations.

Abram starts the dialogue by stating that she feels, after reading Chapter 8, that Bion's work took on themes closely related to Winnicott's late work, albeit in a different language. She notes that both she and Hinshelwood have observed that after Klein's death in 1960, both men seem to be freer in their work and their thought – as if they'd both been released. But while Abram continues to make distinctions, Hinshelwood is concerned to find agreements. He makes the point that both authors had learnt their foundational theories from Klein.

Tensions arise when Abram relates how provoked she feels by Hinshelwood's asking whether Winnicott made any distinction between objective observation and subjective intuition. She feels Hinshelwood has not understood the whole thrust of her work on Winnicott and the emphasis she has put on the infant from the observer's point of view and the infant's subjective experience, which came up in the first book. The dialogue is fruitful, however, because there are further clarifications about distinctions, but Abram has the final word in the dialogue of Part IV by reiterating that focus needs to be placed on the experience of the patient, as Winnicott had emphasised, in order to appreciate fully the infantile layer of human experience.

Part V – "Clinical approach" – aims to address the concepts of countertransference and technique. In this final section of the book, both convergences and divergences are further examined to highlight fundamental differences in the subjects' theory and technique. With reference to a letter from Winnicott to Bion on technique, Winnicott's focus shows to be interpreting the early maternal failures, while Bion illustrates his focus on the "here and now" transference interpretation with a psychotic patient.

In Chapter 9 – "'A sample of the original failure'" – Abram reminds the reader of Winnicott's two analysts: James Strachey, for ten years, followed by Joan Riviere, for five years. This reminder relates to the major influence on Winnicott's developing ideas about the timing of interpretations. Winnicott was particularly exercised by Bion's clinical example given at a Scientific Meeting of the British Psychoanalytical Society. Bion's interpretation to the patient, for Winnicott, was abstract, and as he said at the beginning of his presentation, he would not address the role of the environment in the way in which he interpreted what the patient said during the session.

In Chapter 10 – "Content and process" – Hinshelwood stresses Bion's further evolution in his work on transformations and growth. By 1968, when Winnicott was giving his paper "The use of an object", Bion had left London for Los Angeles and was more interested in writing novels in a search for the meaning of aesthetic "truth". Bion was more focused on the analytic process than the analytic content, and he endorsed the here-and-now transference interpretation, which has remained one of the main techniques of the Kleinian group up until today. This point in Chapter 10 highlights that for Hinshelwood, Bion does indeed address the environment, but it is not the early maternal environment, which Winnicott addresses in his suggestion for an interpretation (Chapter 9); rather, it is the analyst as the here-and-now environment. For Hinshelwood, Bion's interpretation helped the patient become aware of the reality of the weekend break. The difference between these two different ways of interpreting is taken up in the short dialogue.

The dialogue starts with both Abram and Hinshelwood reflecting on their protagonists' late work. It would seem that neither man felt comfortable in the scientific atmosphere of the British Psychoanalytical Society. Abram is still concerned with the meaning of "history" and how it plays out in the transference. This response to the issue of here-and-now interpretations seems to confuse and she asks for the difference between interpreting in the present tense of the transference and interpreting in the here and now. It becomes clear in this dialogue, that while Winnicott was concerned about the patient's experience of the early mother, Bion was not concerned with the psyche's history. He was concerned with what the patient did to the analyst; that is, projective identification.

Further tensions arise when Abram says she feels that Hinshelwood is not answering her questions and that she tends to agree with Winnicott's way of working with the psychotic patient (that is, interpreting the early maternal failure as it is shown in the transference as a "sample of the original failure"). She is reminded of the final dialogue in the first book and how there were tensions about the meaning of the term "illusion". There are further exchanges in this final dialogue which may or may not enlighten the reader about the criticisms of both Winnicott's technique and Bion's. The dialogue concludes, but perhaps not so satisfactorily.

PART I

THE BRITISH PSYCHOANALYTICAL SOCIETY

Chapters 1 and 2 present a general overview and the context in which both Winnicott and Bion evolved their theories. The influence of WW1 had a significant impact on their biographical circumstances and may well have been a major factor in why they chose psychoanalysis as a therapeutic method.

Chapter 1 illustrates Winnicott's standing in the British Psychoanalytical Society (BPaS) and the development of his theories alongside the Kleinian development. Chapter 2 discusses Bion's experience during WW1 and shows how his various attempts to investigate the nature of thinking, and in particular psychoanalytic thinking, that started in his pre-analytic phase.

DOI: 10.4324/9781003382409-2

CHAPTER ONE

Donald Winnicott and the Kleinian development

Jan Abram

D.W.W. (as he used to sign off, in pencil, in the attendance registers for Scientific Meetings of the British Psychoanalytical Society) was born in Plymouth, Devon, on 7 April 1896. Today, Winnicott is known as one of the major conceptual innovators in the history of psychoanalysis during the twentieth century. The primacy of the environment-individual setup is at the core of his formulations and provides psychoanalysis with a new symbolic matrix: that is, the early parent-infant relationship. This particular contribution extends and amplifies the original Freudian Oedipal symbolic matrix. For Winnicott, psychoanalysis constitutes a scientific theory of emotional development and human nature, which is illuminated through the Freudian lens of psychoanalytic practice: "It was only through analysis that I became gradually able to see a baby as a human being. This was really the chief result of my first five years of analysis" (Winnicott, 1989, p. 574). Winnicott's writings invoke the clinical situation and the day-to-day intrapsychic and interpsychic struggle that is demanded of each analyst in clinical work. He is able to convey the ineffability of what it means to be in the continual process of becoming an analyst due to being "on excellent terms with his primary processes" (Milner, 1972, p. 10). "He was first and foremost a psychoanalyst" (Gillespie, 1972, p. 1) who believed that it was essential to

DOI: 10.4324/9781003382409-3

be "firmly rooted in the spirit of the psychoanalytic tradition, rather than the letter of it, if a psychoanalyst wishes to work at the cutting-edge of psychoanalytic discovery" (King, 1972, p 28).

The emphasis on "psychoanalytic discovery" and psychoanalysis as a science was founded on Winnicott's early education at the Leys School, Cambridge, a school well known for the teaching of the sciences. Drawing on Thomas Kuhn's theory of the structure of scientific revolutions, Loparic has argued that Winnicott's debt to Darwin, like those of Freud and Kuhn, showed him that "living things could be studied scientifically, with the corollary that gaps in knowledge and understanding need not scare" (Winnicott, 1996, p. 7), and illustrates how Winnicott's new "exemplar", Kuhn's term for model or paradigm, came about through his clinical discoveries (Loparic, 2013). So, while it is true that Winnicott's prose may be described as poetic, this does not mean that his innovations are more art than science. Winnicott himself always maintained that he did not view the psychoanalytic method as an art. In 1946, in a letter to Ella Sharpe, he writes that he did not agree with psychoanalysis being an art because he felt that psychoanalytic technique is "based on scientific considerations" (Winnicott, 1946).

In a detailed analysis of Winnicott's seminal text "Primitive emotional development", Thomas Ogden observes that "Winnicott does not use language to arrive at conclusions", rather he shares his process of discovery and creates a "non-fiction literature". When reading Winnicott, Ogden writes, there is a "meeting of reader and writing [that] generates an imaginative experience in the medium of language". Ogden proposes that Winnicott's writings are inseparable from the man and the life of his ideas (Ogden, 2001).

Winnicott argues that "dependent or deeply regressed patients can teach the analyst more about early infancy than can be learnt from direct observation of infants, and more than can be learned from contact with mothers who are involved with infants" (Winnicott, 1960). This statement endorses Freud's original argument that innovations in psychoanalysis can only evolve in the context of Freudian clinical methodology, that is, with the analysand on the couch in high-frequency analysis. This is the tried and tested setting in which psychic work can be generated and in which new clinical discoveries can come to light with each different case study. André Green has argued that Winnicott's thought emerged from a close examination of his countertransference in the analytic situation rather than his paediatric work (Green, 1975, 2000). Clinical innovations, therefore, only have value as authentic psychoanalytic advances if they emerge out of the transference-countertransference matrix of the analytic situation.

As I have demonstrated elsewhere (Abram, 2007), Winnicott's capacity to invoke clinical psychoanalytic experience, for both analyst and analysand, gave birth to a distinctive psychoanalytic language. I suggest that it constitutes a "clinical language", which has generated a new theoretical matrix (compare Green on "clinical thinking" (Green, 2005) and Abram, 2022). In other words, Winnicott's clinical innovations, based on scientific investigation and discovery within the analytic setting, are integrated with his conceptual advances. They are of a piece. And this integration was initiated during Winnicott's education at the Leys School:

> As soon as I found Freud and the method he gave us for investigating and for treatment, I was in line with it. This was just like when I was at school and was reading Darwin and suddenly I knew that Darwin was my cup of tea.
>
> (Winnicott, 1989b, p. 574)

Winnicott discovered Freud's work in 1919 at the age of 24. Four years later, after a consultation with Ernest Jones, the founder of the Institute of Psychoanalysis in London, he started analysis with James Strachey, who had just returned from Vienna having had a two year analysis with Sigmund Freud. In 1929, Winnicott started his analytic training at the Institute of Psychoanalysis, only three years after Melanie Klein had come to live and work in London from Berlin.

Freud's clinical method continued to be Winnicott's "cup of tea", and he maintained that "it's an objective way of looking at things...without preconceived notions, which...is science" (Winnicott, Shepherd and Davis, 1989). After a ten-year analysis with James Strachey (1923–1933), who was later the general editor of the *Standard Edition of the Complete Psychological Works of Sigmund Freud*, it is hardly surprising that Winnicott said he always felt that "Freud was in his bones", and he protested that any original ideas he may have "are only valuable as a growth of ordinary Freudian psychoanalytic theory...and would make no sense at all if planted on a world that had not been prepared for it by Freud" (Rodman, 1987, p. 75).

The "learning area" of Melanie Klein

As Winnicott was completing his analysis with James Strachey (circa 1932), he recommended that Winnicott take some consultations from

Melanie Klein, who at the invitation of Ernest Jones had come to live in London from 1926. This was an "important moment" for Winnicott, as he reports, because for some time he had been finding that there was a "certain deficiency" in psychoanalytic theory. During the 1920s, everything had the Oedipus complex at its core, but Winnicott was finding in his paediatric work that babies "could be emotionally ill" long before they reached the stage of the Oedipus complex. This is why Melanie Klein's work on early psychic development was so important for him, and as he said, "Overnight I had changed from being a pioneer into being a student with a pioneer teacher" (Winnicott, 1960, p. 173).

During the 1930s Winnicott benefitted from supervision of his child cases by Melanie Klein during the time when he was treating Klein's son. For a time she was very grateful to Winnicott for his work with her son, and in her letters it can be seen that she also wanted to enlist Winnicott as a follower of her theories. By the time of the beginning of the Controversial Discussions in 1941, Donald Winnicott was named as one of Klein's training analysts. But due to her frustration with him for not submitting work to her prior to a discussion, Klein dropped Winnicott as well as John Rickman. According to Pearl King, this was because they were too "independently minded" to be brought into line by her way of formulating Freudian theories, which, for the Freudians, especially the Viennese Freudians, distorted the classical psychoanalytic paradigm.

Winnicott was "left cold" by the years of scientific discussions between Klein's supporters and Freudians. By 1945, after the apparent conclusion of the theoretical differences when there was a division of training between Kleinians and Freudians, Winnicott presented his paper "Primitive emotional development", which, even now stands as both a theoretical statement and a political one. This paper heralded the beginning of his original formulations, which did not tow any party line, and along with the involvement of many other indigenous analysts of the British Psychoanalytical Society the Independent stream of psychoanalysis was inadvertently inaugurated. It was not until 1968 that an "official" Independent group was formed. To this day, there are three "official" theoretical orientations taught at the British Psychoanalytical Society: Kleinian, Contemporary Freudian, and Independent. A ten-week course in each orientation is mandatory for all psychoanalysts in training. While there are many well-known analysts whose work is associated with the Independent tradition, especially Michael Balint and Ronald Fairbairn, it is Winnicott's clinical paradigm that has become most well known outside of the BPaS.

Recognising a "deficiency" in Freudian theory through his extensive experience as a paediatrician and child analyst certainly motivated Winnicott to reflect on earlier psychic development. He was always grateful for Klein's generosity as a teacher, but gradually he came to see that her formulations of early psychic development did not take enough account of the real woman who was the mother. As we shall see in Chapter 3, Winnicott's quest, as a result of working with Klein, led him to "classify" the environment and its impact on the nascent psyche.

CHAPTER TWO

Wilfred Bion and Klein's schizoid mechanisms

R.D. Hinshelwood

Background

Wilfred Bion, born 1896, came from Imperial India, where his father was an engineer. In Edwardian times, sons were sent back to England to boarding school at the age of eight years. Bion never saw India and his home again after 1905. When he was 19, he joined the army and was put in charge of a unit of the 5th Tank Battalion, fighting battles at Ypres and Amiens. Tanks were experimental weapons and most tank crews died in battle. Bion was fortunate to survive and was nominated for (though not awarded) the Victoria Cross.

He writes of one dreadful occasion (Bion, 1997, pp. 124–127) when he and a young soldier named Sweeting crouched together, "A shell seemed to burst on top of us, and I heard a groan from Sweeting", and the left side of Sweeting's tunic was covered in blood. Bion discovered that Sweeting's left side had been torn away. He was not dead, but he was terrified, and dazed, not realising what had happened to him. Though he tried to look, Bion stopped him: "I pretended to bandage him, but the field dressing was far too small and simply didn't come near to covering the cavity". The boy was saying,

 DOI: 10.4324/9781003382409-4

> "I'm done for, Sir! I'm done for"; [he was] hoping against hope I would contradict him. This I did, telling him it was nothing – but his eyes were already glazing over, and it was clear that death was even then upon him. In the last moments he kept trying to cough, but the wind came from his side instead, and he kept trying to ask why he couldn't cough.
> (Bion, 1997, p. 131)

Bion's description is painful to read, and he described the incident a number of times in various autobiographical attempts until the 1970s (published posthumously). His daughter Parthenope noted there was "hardly any emotional or intellectual elaboration" (Bion Talamo, 1997, p 309). As Bion wrote in his diaries of the war: "I never recovered from the survival of the Battle of Amiens" (Bion, 1997, p 209); and much later, in the 1970s: "Oh yes, I died on August 8th 1918" (Bion, 1982, p 265).

He had some psychotherapy afterwards while a student at Queens College, Oxford, in 1920, where he studied history and philosophy. But by the mid-1920s he was aiming at training as a psychoanalyst and went to medical school (University College Hospital, London). There he was impressed when he worked for a surgeon, Wilfred Trotter, who was a long-term friend of Ernest Jones and was Freud's surgeon after Freud came to England in 1938. Bion said of Trotter that listened with an unassumed interest, "as if the patient's contributions flowed from the fount of knowledge itself" (Bion, 1985, p 36). Bion says it took him years of experience to learn that the patient's story is in fact of overriding importance. His career was dominated all the way through by an emphasis on listening and, indeed, the need to grasp how we can "know" the experience that another is relating to us.

At some point Bion had another psychotherapy session, with J.A. Hadfield, the director of training at the Tavistock Clinic, and in 1932 he went to the clinic to train as a psychotherapist. The clinic was home to British eclecticism (Brown, 1964), and at the time deeply disapproved of by the British Psychoanalytical Society. He was appointed to the staff in 1934, attended Jung's (1968) Tavistock Lectures in 1935 (accompanied on one occasion by his patient Samuel Beckett), but clearly began to feel dissatisfied and decided to train at the Institute of Psychoanalysis, starting a training analysis with John Rickman in 1938.

Rickman (1891–1951), a Quaker, had worked for the Friends' War Victims Relief Service in Russia during World War 1, and developed an anthropological interest. He was personally acquainted with W.H.R Rivers and Geza Roheim. Rickman had an analysis with Freud in the

1920s, supplemented a few years later by an analysis with Ferenczi, and in the late 1930s by sessions with Melanie Klein. His analysis of Bion was interrupted in 1939 by the war and was never resumed. Instead, Rickman became something of mentor for Bion (Vonofakos and Hinshelwood, 2012; Hinshelwood, 2018), and with Rickman's psychosocial interest and Bion's eclecticism at the time, they engaged in experiments with groups in military psychiatry in the British Army.

Bion was married in 1940, to Betty Jardine, a film-star, but tragically she died after the birth of their first child, in early 1945. In that year, immediately after the war ended, Bion started an analysis with Melanie Klein with a view to psychoanalytic training, and he became a member of the society in 1950.

The paranoid-schizoid position

By the time he became a psychoanalyst, Bion was a significant and celebrated authority on group therapy (Bion, 1961), although he had revised his view of his fundamental concepts of groups as he became a psychoanalyst (Bion, 1952). He joined Klein's inner circle of colleagues in the early 1950s, exploiting Klein's (1946) description of splitting and the schizoid mechanisms in experimental analyses of psychotic states. He specialised in the thought disorder of schizophrenia (while Rosenfeld investigated the disorders of identity and identification, and Segal discovered the underlying problem of symbol-formation in psychosis). From around 1958 to 1959, Bion's interest in thinking began to be applied to the scientific thinking of psychoanalysts. His philosophical background (basically Kantian) began to be applied to psychoanalysis and to psychoanalysts' claims for their scientific results. In 1960 Klein died, and it was as if the obligation of being tied to her was released, and in the 1960s he thought deeply about the epistemology of psychoanalysis. His discovery of the container-contained model in the late 1950s relied on Klein's understanding of the very early processes of projection and introjection of experiences, and indeed of parts of the self. This theory of personal development is a partially interpersonal accomplishment, though deeply interfered with by unconscious anxieties and phantasies of the schizoid kind (Bion, 1959).

Following Klein, Bion accepted that there is an ego from birth with some sort of coherent boundary. However, that coherence is experienced as fragile and easily seen as under attack from various sources. Central at this time of the very earliest development is the anxiety about one's own survival (persecutory anxiety), which only slowly evolves towards anxiety about harming a loved other (depressive anxiety) (Klein, 1935).

Not least of the defences against persecutory anxiety are the primitive processes of projection, introjection, and identification, which split the ego itself. As Klein had said, the patient's destructiveness can turn from the object towards a destructiveness towards the self. Such a self-destructiveness is aimed at coping with the major anxiety. Of course, the hypothesised splitting off of experiences that carry persecutory anxiety can promote further anxiety about the incoherence and destruction of the self, a cyclical process which in extreme cases results in the severely split-up condition of psychosis (Bion, 1957).

However, with the support of reality and the increasing awareness of others and their stability the ego can introject a greater sense of coherence and survival and learn the reality of dependence on those external objects (a step towards what is known as the depressive position). For much of his career, Bion's ambition was to understand how that important relation with reality is interfered with. He followed Freud's emphasis on the importance of the reality principle and Klein's on the envy of objects depended on. He was adept at understanding the splitting processes and interpreting the deeply splintered state of the ego existing as a series of "part-objects".

Summary

Both our protagonists' development in their early lives was probably quite rigidly defined by English Edwardian culture. Winnicott seemed to move relatively smoothly from his WW1 experiences, despite having experienced trauma during his service in WW1, to his lifelong career, while Bion was more troubled and took probably 20 years to fully decide on his career path into psychoanalysis.

Both were highly influenced by Melanie Klein, although by different phases of her career – Winnicott by her discovery of the play technique with children, and Bion by her subsequent interest in the incoherence of the ego and the schizoid defences. And perhaps as a result, they came to emphasise different aspects of her object-relations approach. Winnicott advanced the importance of the parent infant relationship and its influence on the individual's intrapsychic dynamics, while Bion emphasised listening in the clinical setting and the nature of the connection between self and other – intuition and the container-contained model. The main point of agreement between them concerns sensitivity to the analyst's own experience of being with the patient. And they both acknowledged how indebted they were to Melanie Klein and accepted the importance of the *pre*-Oedipal development of children.

However, they disagree most profoundly on the primitive mechanisms Klein described in 1946. Winnicott placed far more emphasis on the actual psychic quality of the mothering an infant receives and pre-empted Klein's paper with his own in 1945 on the "primitive" experiences an infant struggles with. Bion very explicitly adopted Klein's schizoid mechanisms, exploring their value relative to psychotic states and psychotic parts of everyone's personality.

Table 1 Context: The British Psychoanalytical Society

Winnicott	*Bion*
1. Close examination of the countertransference	1. The emphasis is on listening with an unassumed interest
2. Regressed patients teach us more about early infancy than direct observation	2. Experiments with groups in military psychiatry were a strong influence
3. The environment-individual setup has primacy	3. Bion evolved the container-contained model from projective identification
4. Winnicott had many consultations with Melanie Klein	4. Klein's splitting and the schizoid mechanisms became basic theorisation
5. He was a pioneer student with a pioneer teacher	5. He explored psychoanalysis as a form of scientific thinking
6. Mother's psyche is the external environment	6. He accepted an ego-boundary from birth
	7. Self-destructive splitting was a founding assumption
	8. He was dissatisfied with eclecticism

Dialogue

Jan Abram: To think of an eight-year-old being sent so far away from everything that was familiar, to a boarding school in a foreign country, is heartbreaking and shocking, even though I am fully aware of this tradition and how it continues in many countries of the world. I was struck by how you presented this piece of Bion's history in just three short sentences, Bob. It made me wonder about his mother. Where was she? It also reminded me that Winnicott was also sent away to a boarding school. But he was already 14 years of age when that occurred, and the school was in Cambridge, which is only about three hundred miles from his hometown of Plymouth. Winnicott was born a year before Bion, even though Bion did not qualify as an analyst until 15 years after Winnicott had qualified.

You also took us rather quickly from the eight-year-old Bion to a time eleven years later. The nineteen-year-old Bion took on huge responsibilities during WW1. To oversee an army unit battling in Belgium and France was highly dangerous and must have been terrifying. The account of his witnessing his fellow soldier who had been severely wounded yet was still alive and talking to Bion was moving and, again, shocking. It's impressive to hear that Bion wrote about this in his later years and that his daughter noted that he wrote with little emotional elaboration. Yet, it would seem that he needed to write about it. Despite that, he says he never recovered from surviving the Battle of Amiens, which suggests he suffered from survivor guilt.

Winnicott also suffered from survivor guilt, it would seem, after WW1, according to his second wife, Clare Winnicott (Winnicott, 1978). As he was born in Plymouth, he signed up for the Navy at 19 and was posted to a destroyer. Evidently he was the only doctor on the ship – a medical probationer officer – although he was not fully qualified, as he interrupted his medical studies at Jesus College, Cambridge, in the final nine months before WW1 ended. Inevitably, like Bion, Winnicott witnessed a huge amount of carnage on the destroyer, and as the sole medical officer we can only imagine that Bion's experience of Sweeting dying like that was something that Winnicott would be familiar with. He did not write about it directly, although at the heart of his work is the notion of "survival of the object".

So, from the very beginning of your chapter, we are confronted with a picture of trauma due to specific life events. Being sent away to school at such a young age, never to return, would certainly traumatise any young child. But we don't have a picture of what his early environment was like. Did he know what it was like to have a truly good mother, or had he already spent much of his early life being looked after by a nanny? I wonder about this because it is this kind of detail that is relevant to the theories both authors came to formulate – Winnicott on holding and Bion on the container-contained. We'll be referring to these concepts I'm sure as we continue our dialogues for each part.

Bion knew he was traumatised but we don't really know to what extent. Perhaps you know more. I wonder whether he realised he was already traumatised when he joined the army. I have the impression it was courageous of him to seek therapy when studying at Oxford. At that time a "stiff upper lip" was more in keeping with his class and culture.

Wilfred Trotter was an important influence in Winnicott's training at Barts, emphasising the importance of history taking. John Rickman was also one of the analysts that Winnicott quoted in his early work, and when Rickman died in 1950, Winnicott took over the analysis of one of Rickman's patients, Masud Khan, who had been in supervision for his first training case with Winnicott. Pearl King had also been in analysis with John Rickman when he died in 1950, and she then went into analysis with her supervisor, Marion Milner (Winnicott, 1986, pp. 123–127). This appears to have been the solution to Rickman's sudden death for both Khan and King.

Bion seems to have been fostered by Melanie Klein and her supporters right from the beginning of his training. You point out that he was already a well-known figure and an authority on group therapy. Bion focused on groups and schizophrenia while Winnicott's interest was in finding and appreciating the ordinary good mother because it was to mothers he "so deeply needed to speak" (Winnicott, [1957] in Winnicott, 1986).

I imagine it might have been difficult for Winnicott to witness Bion being in analysis with Klein and being applauded by her and her staunch supporters such as Hannah Segal and Betty Joseph. Despite having his own following from 1945 onwards and also being well known outside the society for his work with families, Winnicott, it is reported, always felt disappointed that Melanie Klein did not afford him a real dialogue, for example the way we have been attempting since 2014. Winnicott became president of the society for the first time in 1956, when Bion was still a fairly newly qualified analyst and not yet a training analyst.

From what you say, Bion was taken with Melanie Klein's formulations on early anxieties. I assume you mean that he agreed with her that her formulation of the paranoid-schizoid position depicted the mind of all infants at the beginning of life. I remember that in 2014 this was one of the first theories we discussed. I baulked at the idea that babies are murderous from the beginning of life. Winnicott did not accept this formulation, as you're aware, and we discussed that in our first book of this series (Abram and Hinshelwood, 2018).

To summarise for this opening of the first dialogue let me outline what interests me after reading your chapter.

1. Both Winnicott and Bion suffered trauma related to their family environment. Bion was younger when he was sent far away to school,

never to return, so it follows that he was more traumatised. Winnicott, being seven years older when sent away to school, had benefitted from more years in the family and was presumably more emotionally equipped to deal with the separation. We can see evidence of his ability to deal with separation in his letters to his mother and sisters (interestingly, his father was never included in these letters).

2. Both Winnicott and Bion suffered some kind of war trauma as a result of witnessing terrible wounds to their fellow sailors and soldiers – carnage and death. These events are de facto traumatic, but we know that depending on the strength of the ego in earlier development, the severity would depend on the depth of trauma suffered later. I would imagine that Bion, again, suffered more than Winnicott because his ego was less developed. This is a hypothesis based on psychoanalytic theory. Nevertheless, Winnicott was most certainly traumatised. As a very inexperienced and not-yet-qualified medic he presumably did his best to save many sailors who were seriously wounded, and even with full qualifications he would not have been able to save everyone.
3. It seems clear that both men suffered from what we often refer to as survivor guilt. At one level, individuals are relieved they are not dead, but inevitably this comes at an emotional cost because of a deep sense of guilt that the siblings die while you survived and lived.

This leads me on to reflect on the concept of trauma. Quite early in his work Winnicott formulated his particular theory of trauma. He did not refer specifically to the trauma of war but rather to the earliest trauma, that is, birth trauma (Winnicott, 1949; Abram, 2021).

Therefore, for Winnicott, the paranoid-schizoid position constitutes early trauma. In fact the characteristics of the paranoid-schizoid position demonstrated a clear picture of what Winnicott came to refer to as an "environmental deficiency disease". In other words, the features are caused by a failing holding environment and do not illustrate a universal fact at the beginning of life (see Glossary for a definition of "holding"). This particular difference in our protagonists' perspectives on early psychic life highlights fundamentally different basic assumptions which inevitably lead to clinical approaches that are different and possibly incompatible.

Robert D. Hinshelwood: I think you bring out well the impact of WW1 on both Bion and Winnicott. In fact, no one in that generation could have avoided being seriously affected. Bion, so far as we know, was very attached to his ayah (Hindi for nanny), and there has always been considerable speculation as to how much the ayah's culture left a trace of Eastern culture in Bion's occasional turn to mysticism. He is known to have had Alan Watts' *The Way of Zen* in his library and to have made a margin comment or two. However, Bion cannot have been alone in Edwardian times in being torn from his family in the empire at the age of eight or fourteen. This was a common experience, and English culture has tended to see the upbringing of children as training rather than as nurturing. I am sure this is the common background for both Bion and Winnicott. How they dealt with it is very different indeed. Winnicott, already in medical training, pursued that career immediately after the war and became one of the very first paediatricians, and no doubt followed a (conscious or unconscious) enquiry into childhood health and psychology.

Bion however, was adrift for a decade until he decided to return to university and train as a doctor. To my mind, Bion was indeed traumatised by his war experience. His repeated descriptions of the Sweeting incident seem like the textual equivalent of the typical flashbacks of "war neurosis", as it was called (Ferenczi et al, 1921), or PTSD as it is now called in sterile diagnostic terminology. Maybe your term "survivor guilt" is better psychoanalytically as it has a psychodynamic quality rather than using the objectifying style of psychology and psychiatry.

One important issue is trauma. It is not clear that Bion or Kleinians have a concept of trauma in the same way as more classical schools, including Winnicott. For Kleinians trauma *is* the paranoid-schizoid position; it is the belief one is being destroyed, whatever sense an infant can make of it. And indeed a lot of Bion's early work as a psychoanalyst suggests to me that he was trying to rediscover that deep sense of being destroyed. I would say his descriptions of mental fragmentation (see Bion, 1958) and the picture of a mind exploding into infinite space (see Bion, 1970, ch. 2) are just such attempts at capturing the primitive experience.

Those descriptions and the repeated autobiographical descriptions of the horrors of WW1 seem like the equivalent of the flashbacks that typify PTSD. He referred later in his work to catastrophic change and to caesuras, using Freud to try to draw together disparate bits on either side of the caesura. But remarkably, it seems Bion did recover from that experience.

Bion did not work with children, and as you say, he came to psychoanalysis through inventing an approach to groups, especially those in the army (in the Second World War). Instead, Bion had his own children. A narrative that has always struck me as plausible is that the ghastly way in which the children of the English upper classes were brought up ensured that when the psychoanalytic society in Britain was formed, it had a persisting interest in the experience of children (the child in themselves, no doubt). This would have prompted the adulation that Klein received when she moved to London in 1926, being known by then as a pioneer in understanding children. In addition, she herself would, I think, have been enormously interested in this rare paediatrician. And although Winnicott did not qualify as a psychoanalyst until 1934, at the same time the paediatrician in him must have been very drawn to her. In fact, Winnicott, I believe, sought Klein as his second analyst. Klein did not agree, because she wished at the time to ask Winnicott to take her own child Erich into treatment with him.

Something happened in the early 1940s, it seems, which appears to have been instigated by Winnicott when he took up a series of disagreements with Klein's views, at first notably via his presuming that Klein neglected the actual external object in reality (a dispute that began to smoulder in the British Psychoanalytical Society in the late 1930s). Klein herself, never very good at engaged debate, did perhaps drop Winnicott, and from 1945 turned her attention to Bion (as well as to Herbert Rosenfeld and Hannah Segal). It could certainly have struck chords in both Bion and Winnicott concerning the sort of exile they had both suffered as children exported to boarding school. However, at this time Bion seemed to be the slightly perplexed winner of a sibling struggle. It could then seem, from a Kleinian point of view, that this was a rageful experience for Winnicott which he could never quite grasp.

As you say, clearly Winnicott and Bion put the devastating violence and survival anxieties of WW1 behind them in very different ways, and at a very different pace. Bion's trajectory into psychoanalysis is complex, taking more than a quarter of a century after the end of the war, and entailed his apprenticeship as a therapist at the Tavistock, where he was influenced by Jung, an influence he seems to have mostly rejected, turning to an analysis with John Rickman in 1938 and then finding an enormous creativity in being able to convert his analyst (after 1939) into a kind of mentor (Hinshelwood, 2018). He then resumed his formal psychoanalytic training in 1945: he went to Klein as his analyst, some six months after the further tragedy, the loss of his wife in childbirth.

I think I want to emphasise a couple of important observations from these two papers that start this part of the book:

1. Your notion of both intrapsychic and interpsychic dimensions seems important to bear in mind, as it is a hallmark of both Winnicott and

Bion's work, if not perhaps of the whole of British psychoanalysis. Today we hear so much of inter-personal, inter-subjective, relational forms of psychoanalysis which often seem to seriously downplay the intrapsychic, which is above all the specific psychoanalytic contribution. And as we shall see as we proceed, Bion and Winnicott were in general agreement, though rivalrous and diverging on how to couple the intrapsychic with a necessary respect for the reality principle.

2. The second interesting thing that strikes me is the sense of a homogeneous whole you give to Winnicott's work, because this contrasts so strikingly with Bion's constant restlessness in his clinical thinking about individual patients and with his diverse reading in philosophy, literature, and aesthetics, and even in mysticism (there was, incidentally, a medieval saint in France called Saint Bion). This gives such a different view of their separate journeys.

I wanted to write a further point about the intra-, interpsychic matrix which both Bion and Winnicott pursued. It is probably true that Winnicott and Klein both grounded their understanding of babies in the babies' *experience* of the external mother. Where Winnicott wanted to go beyond Klein was in understanding the mother's experience and her psychodynamics, which Klein more or less refused to do. It is then questionable whether, in a psychoanalytic treatment of a patient, one can truly engage in an understanding of the mother (who, of course, is not present) as the external object that Winnicott prescribed.

Bion was, it seems to me, on a similar track to Winnicott, rather than to Klein here, and perhaps he was led by Winnicott (in fact, I think one could read a lot of Bion's ideas as unacknowledged responses to issues that Winnicott highlighted first). As we go on, I think we will consider the specific way in which Bion felt he could advance on Winnicott's somewhat objective (rather than experiential) analysis of "mother".

J.A.: So Bion's early attachment figure seems to have been his ayah. This would suggest that his mother may not have breast fed him or had any great closeness to him. It makes me wonder about Bion's transference to Melanie Klein, and Winnicott's too of course. But I'm still wondering what happened to Bion's mother. Does he never speak about her? And how many siblings did he have?

Winnicott was the youngest of three children. In a large family portrait, in Rodman's biography, he is in the middle of the photo looking uncomfortable and not so happy. He looks as if he is between two and three years of age (Rodman, 2003: 145). But his letters from boarding school to his sisters and mother are always warm and informative.

You do acknowledge that the issue of trauma on a personal level is wholly relevant to both Winnicott and Bion. You seem to intimate that there is no theory of trauma in Kleinian theory – rather it is subsumed in the theory of the paranoid-schizoid position. I wonder if you could elaborate on this? This concept is one of the basic assumptions that are fundamentally different between Winnicott and Bion. You refer to Bion's early papers, suggesting that through his work he was "trying to re-discover that deep sense of being destroyed"; do you mean due to his earliest unconscious experience, which was reinforced by boarding school and then his time served as a soldier in WW1?

Does Bion, like Klein, believe that the infantile position – the first few weeks of life – is de facto traumatic? Is this why there is no need for a theory of trauma? The Kleinian position, and therefore Bion's, seems to suggest that every single baby will be traumatised at the start of life because the paranoid-schizoid position is a universal fact. Could you elaborate further, Bob, on how you understand this difference about such a fundamental concept? This was one of the reasons that the Freudians were so enraged with Klein's thinking during the Controversial Discussions, wasn't it? Does it mean that emotional development is all about "recovering" from the psychotic state of mind in the earliest hours, days, and weeks?

You're right, Bob, when you point out that Melanie Klein, according to various sources, was interested in Winnicott when he sought consultation for his child cases with her in the early 1930s. There is correspondence published in Rodman's biography and Grosskurth's biography of Klein which highlights how grateful she was for his work with her son and how much she wished to enlist his further help in 1941 when she was worried about Eric (Rodman, 2003, p. 116). She and Joan Riviere, who was Winnicott's second analyst after Strachey, evidently tried to tell Winnicott that he did not understand what they were saying about early infancy. In his letter of 1956 to Riviere, Winnicott wrote that when he talked to Melanie Klein about her statement on early infancy he felt as if he "were talking about colour to the colour-blind". He thought that she showed no evidence of acknowledging the part the mother plays at the very beginning.

I think what Winnicott meant is that in Klein's theory there is no theorising of the mother. The focus is on what is innate, that is, the paranoid-schizoid position and endowment. The mother's role is to mitigate the terrors of the beginning, but the details of her intervention are not formulated into a theory.

And isn't this where Bion comes in? He fills in the gap in Kleinian theory and does formulate the mother's role when he refers to the importance of the mother's reverie in containing the infant's terrors of dying. This seems to me to be the advance in the Kleinian paradigm.

Winnicott was disappointed and hurt by the end of his analysis with Joan Riviere (circa 1941), as can be seen in the excerpt above of his letter to Riviere, which is related also to the comments he received from both her and Melanie about his paper "On the observation of infants in a set situation", which he delivered to the British Psychoanalytical Society in 1942 (Winnicott, 1941; Rodman, 2003). By the beginning of the Controversial Discussions in 1942, Winnicott, although named as a Kleinian analyst, was already moving away from her theories because his contribution was not valued by Klein and her followers.

But back to Bion. It must have been very traumatising for Bion, on top of his losses during the war, when his first wife died in childbirth at the end of the war. To go into analysis only six months after this tragedy must have been helpful and necessary, to say the least, I can imagine.

Let me respond to the two observations you make. The first on the notion of the intrapsychic and interpsychic and the second on your response to my rendering of the homogenous whole, as you put it, of Winnicott's work.

I think that there is a particular emphasis on the intrapsychic–interpsychic dimension of the transference specific to British analysis. Often in clinical seminars it is not obvious whether the analyst is an Independent, Kleinian, or Contemporary Freudian. The distinctions are only obvious during a theoretical discussion of a case; for example when reading a publication. I think this is where we probably work in a similar vein as we have already discovered. I remember at the Warsaw conference on Winnicott and Bion in 2017 we found much accord in how we reflected on clinical work.

The relationist school and interpersonalists in general highly esteem Winnicott's and Bion's work and are very well read in their work. But often, it seems to me, they have a different way of applying the theories in their clinical encounters and, at times, take their work rather too literally.

I'm not sure I would call the whole of Winnicott's trajectory homogenous. However, it is true that his disagreement with Klein focused on the crucial factor that the real mother's psyche has an impact on the infant's nascent psyche, that is, the reality of her interpsychic communications. Winnicott's epiphany in 1942 – "There's no such thing as a baby" – continued to evolve as a concept up until his very late work, in which he was very clear that without the reality of a dedicated mother at the beginning, the infant would have no chance of developing into a healthy adult.

So, his work from 1942 up till his death in early 1971 can be seen to evolve with a focus on the mother's contribution to her infant, seeing this as key to her contribution to society.

I wonder if you're indicating that Bion was less stable due to being so traumatised? His late work is often criticised by the London Kleinians, is it not? And yet perhaps his way of working when he left London might have been a response to the Kleinian culture in London. Can you say more about this? Winnicott, despite being disappointed and hurt, continued to thrive within his own collegial group and was totally dedicated to committee work with the British Society. He was its president on two occasions (in 1956 and 1965).

I have a different view to you, Bob, when you point out that both Winnicott and Klein "grounded their understanding of babies in the baby's experience of the external mother". When I read Klein I am much more aware of the emphasis on the baby's internal world and find it hard to have a sense of what the baby is making of the mother. By contrast, and we discussed this in our first book, in reading Winnicott I have a sense of the dyadic dynamic between the newborn and mother, of how essential it is for her to "adapt" to infantile needs and the extent to which the infant will benefit from the experience of feeling like god at the very beginning.

I suppose what you mean about Bion being on a "similar track" to Winnicott is that he started to reflect on the important role the mother had to play in early psychic development. Although this might be true, Bion did not change his mind about the infant being psychotic at the start as a result of the paranoid-schizoid position. I think this is what became clear to me in the International Psychoanalytic Association (IPA) webinar we participated in on 11 April 2021 when we discussed the clinical work of Bion and Winnicott's letter to him (Abram and Hinshelwood, 2021). Did I get this right, that Bion's view would be that we all have a psychotic and non-psychotic part of our personalities? This does not hold in Winnicott's theory, but I will refer to that more in Chapter 4.

It does seem clear that Bion became more interested in the mother's role, which crystallises in his theory of the container-contained (Bion, 1962a). And in Part II of this book we will be looking at working with children and groups when we discuss the two very different first professions of each man, Winnicott the paediatrician and Bion, whose early therapeutic interest was in groups and the psychosocial.

R.D.H: You ask several questions which I will try to address, and I want to make a couple of points about Bion's approach to clinical practice at the beginning of his psychoanalytic work. Firstly, Bion says little about his mother – or his ayah. He had, I believe, a younger sister, who he may not have known well, having left the family aged eight.

I suspect, Bion might have been more disturbed psychiatrically, if that is significant. I do think he was looking desperately for stability in a world of experiences which felt fragmented and fragmenting. Does this mean we should take him less seriously, or does it mean, in the right circumstances (which I think he had), he could give us a special insight into this loss of self and being? I would say the latter, but with a cautious recognition of the former.

Now, the intractable point about the paranoid-schizoid position, which Bion accepted all through his career to the end: he was interested in the internal world as a society of "little people", as Klein called internal objects, even in the three novels he wrote in the mid-to-late '70s before he died in 1979. And his "group" inside was made up of internalised others and parts of himself, implying he solidly agreed with the fundamental experiences of introjection and splitting of the ego. Both those "mechanisms" (or phantasies) are central to the paranoid-schizoid position, together with projective identification, which implies the projection of one or another of those little figures as templates, as it were, to see in other persons he encountered in the external world. He never gave this up.

It is a more or less innate way of proceeding psychically from birth. Part of the endowment of objects that inhabit the world inside the boundary of the ego is terrifying, at least at first. I think that Bion is completely Freudian in the sense that he would say there were two initial states of mind from the beginning – a blissful satisfied state, post-feeding for instance, and also (and this is where we find a disagreement between Winnicott and Klein-Bion) another state of unsatisfied need or even pain; and perhaps at the beginning the infant cannot distinguish between unsatisfied need and actual harmful pain. The infant's resource is then the opposite of bliss. I think Freud starts here with this kind of binary response as an innate endowment. I find it hard to follow Winnicott, who you convey did not see this binary endowment – or if he did he couldn't or wouldn't see the states as binary opposites. And indeed, it is not really conceivable that any of us were brought up with the mothering that never allowed the opposite of bliss. As you say, this evolved into a theory of containing, circa 1956–1957.

Now Bion, following Klein (and not Freud), regarded these two states – bliss and its terrifying opposite – in a specific way. He did not switch to saying, "My goodness what was mother doing?" Instead, he kept to his interest in the psychoanalytic focus explicitly on the *infant's* way of experiencing what mother was doing. Instead of switching, like Freud, to instinctual energy and its vicissitudes and opposites, Bion tried to make sense of the infant's experience *as the infant did*. That is, the infant has no idea of the real external mother, or of "the reality of her interpsychic communications", as you put it, only of an object that satisfies and an object that doesn't. The infant does not have the perceptual or conceptual resources to understand the actual mother. Instead, he only has the resources endowed at the beginning (of course, he picks up new skills for understanding his experiences very quickly over the first days and weeks). At first, the needs and their satisfaction/frustration are seen in intentional ways. Some "thing" aims to cause the experience, bliss or horror. If the experience is a bodily sensation (we presume mostly they must be so at the beginning), then the "thing" is something inside his body, inside his ego boundary, that does this to him, bliss or terror. Gradually, as his distance receptors (especially eyes) become useable, he will experience these "objects" outside as well as inside him. I do not think that Bion was at variance with this conception of early life at all. But we know Winnicott was.

I think Bion and Winnicott (and Klein) would agree that everything in the future depends on the rough balance between primary satisfactions and the primary frustrations. The point about trauma is that trauma is the terror in the state of frustration, which is what we experience in horror films, which still fascinate us into old age because they stem from the earliest of terrors. There is no real sense in which this horrifying terror resembles the actually external mother.

Now, one detail that Bion added, a very important detail and a complex one, is that he thought that in the worst situations there is no coping with the terror. Maybe this equates with Winnicott describing the state of frustration as being prolonged for more than the child can cope with. This is so explicit in Winnicott's (1963) "Theory of the parent-infant relationship", where frustration for too long leads to a loss of the ego – he called it the loss of the continuity-of-being. I think actually Bion was on exactly the same lines, but describing exactly, in 1956 ("On hallucinations"), more precise details of how the ego disintegrates. A patient cannot stand the frustration (probably the gap between the sessions), so his first "act" is to fragment his own awareness by splitting up his visual awareness and attacking the bad object (the patient's experience of Bion) by forcing the fragments into Bion. And then, in the patient's experience, the actual external Bion will feel these horror objects and will reproject them back into the patient when he arrives next day. Then, finally, as he lies down on the couch, the patient deposits them in the corner of the room. I have perhaps condensed this story for purposes of comprehension, but it displays the experience of the mind as reduced to concrete, physical bits and pieces – by the reactive hate in the patient who attacks himself, specifically his awareness of his reality – which are then moved from one to the other of the two parties in the room. This patient was of course in an acute state of active psychosis.

Bion describes it as typical in some degree of the paranoid-schizoid position, but then it can repeat in a vicious circle. As John Steiner described:

> One such situation arises if persecutory anxiety becomes excessive, which may leave the individual feeling that his very survival is at risk. Such a threat may paradoxically lead to further fragmentation, which involves minute splitting and violent projection of the fragments.
>
> (Steiner, 1993, p. 30)

So, the defence of attacking one's own perception (the splitting and fragmenting of the ego) leads to an increased sense of going to pieces in a violent way, which leads to a further round of persecuting survival anxiety and of the vicious circle and ultimately frank psychosis – or as Winnicott says, a loss of the continuity of being.

I will now write the two main points I want to make about Bion's work as he came into his formal psychoanalytic training in 1945. From his pre-psychoanalytic years, Bion absorbed the idea of intuition, which he applied to psychoanalytic practice all through his career, from his work with groups to his latest work in the late 1970s. I also want to indicate a second point – Bion's insistence that finding out about the patient's unconscious is a collaboration between analyst and patient.

Bion started out at university straight after WW1 studying history and philosophy. He made friends with a young don, dean of Queens College, Oxford, at the time, who was a budding scholar specialising in Immanuel Kant (and later became an Oxford professor of philosophy). One of Kant's prime principles (one that I can understand) is "Thinking without intuition is empty, and intuition without concepts is blind". We don't make something of the world outside by seeing it as it actually is. We make something of the world by using the ideas and templates we already have in mind, our pre-conceptions. This is a model Bion explored extensively in the 1960s as a new epistemology for psychoanalysis. For instance, he says about the work of analysis, one looks for the following: "The coming together of a sudden precipitating intuition, of a mass of apparently unrelated incoherent phenomena which are thereby given coherence and meaning" (Bion, 1967, p. 168).

Bion frequently uses the term "intuition", and he may have blended his Kantian notion with the more ordinary notion used by Jung (who Bion encountered in the 1930s). But throughout his life, "intuition" seemed to indicate a kind of direct knowledge of another mind. Bion really tried to get into the details and the elements of this kind of mental operation. He contrasted intuition with what he called sensuous experience:

> The physician is dependent on realization of sensuous experience in contrast with the psycho-analyst whose dependence is on experience that is not sensuous. The physician can see and touch and smell. The realizations with which a psycho-analyst deals cannot be seen or touched; anxiety has no shape or colour, smell or sound. For convenience, I propose to use the term "intuit" as a parallel in the psychoanalyst's domain to the physician's use of "see", "touch", "smell", and "hear".
>
> (Bion, 1970, p. 7)

In the same book he complained that words and verbal formulations have evolved to give expression to sensuous experience and that this has handicapped psychoanalysis in dealing with the much more direct grasp of experiences. For Bion, the direct transfer of experience from person to person was admirably grasped by Klein's description of projective identification. Projective identification is a non-verbal, non-symbolic communication which impacts on the other rather than informing the other.

Another point concerns responsibility, which again preceded his formal psychoanalytic training. It was especially apparent in his work in military psychiatry in WW2. He engaged his ward of soldiers as a commander sending his men out to do battle. He pointed to the enemy, and they fired the guns. His interpretive work was not an authoritarian airing of the analyst's opinions and theories – it was a joint responsibility of the analyst's and the patient's conscious minds together. As Frances Tustin wrote about her analysis with Bion in the 1960s:

> He provoked me to think for myself – to have a mind of my own. He did this by asking challenging questions and by making unexpected remarks rather than by imposing a rigid interpretive scheme on what I said and did. In so doing, he made me think about what was happening to me in my own terms
>
> (Tustin, 1981, p 176)

His patient, Frances Tustin, stressed Bion's insistence that she use her own terms and think for herself.

Intuition and joint responsibility were hallmarks of Bion's clinical approach from the beginning of his career. This formed a striking continuity and contrasted with the many theoretical ideas he picked up and dropped.

PART II

ANALYTIC WORK WITH CHILDREN AND GROUPS

Chapters 3 and 4 address the very different first professions of Winnicott and Bion. Winnicott was a doctor who specialised in paediatrics, while Bion studied history and philosophy, beginning as a schoolteacher, but later came to medicine and psychotherapy as the route to becoming a psychoanalyst.

Early on Winnicott observed the important role of the environment in psychic development emanating from his personal analysis alongside his paediatric practice. Bion's influence stretched way beyond psychoanalysis, starting from his initial university studies and his psychosocial focus acquired from the Tavistock Clinic, and then, when he started his work as a psychoanalyst, expanding to take in the intense anxieties of psychotic self-destructiveness, following Klein (1946), and wider reading in the philosophy of science and, eventually, aesthetics.

DOI: 10.4324/9781003382409-5

CHAPTER THREE

Babies and their families

Jan Abram

Foundations (1919–1934)

In a talk he gave to medical students in 1970, months before he died, Winnicott told them he had never wanted to be anything other than a doctor (Winnicott, 1970). By all accounts he seemed to have made this decision at the age of 16 when he was boarding at the Leys School in Cambridge. He matriculated to the University of Cambridge and resided at Jesus College in 1914, and only two years later started to treat patients who were wounded from WW1 when several colleges were converted into temporary military hospitals. Many of his friends had enlisted and subsequently died, and according to Clare Winnicott, his second wife, he was profoundly affected and "always felt he had a responsibility to live for those who died as well as for himself" (Winnicott,, C 1978, p. 27). As a medical student who was assisting in treating patients wounded on the battlefield, Winnicott was exempt from conscription, but in 1917 he wanted to enlist in the Royal Navy (perhaps the obvious choice, having been brought up in Plymouth). He was posted to a destroyer as a surgeon-probationer. Just before the end of WW1, Winnicott entered the medical school of St. Bartholomew's Hospital, London, to complete his medical training, qualifying in 1920.

DOI: 10.4324/9781003382409-6

On his return from his service on the destroyer, Winnicott was disturbed that he was not remembering his dreams. He sought help from a well-known medical bookshop in London, and this seeking, as if he recognised it as a symptom, resulted in discovering psychoanalysis. Freud's book *The Interpretation of Dreams* was first published in 1900, and the first English translation was published in 1913. It was probably this latter translation that Winnicott read. For a while, psychoanalysis became his "hobby", as he wrote to his sister Violet, but soon he was planning to train as an analyst beyond his medical training. He qualified in 1920 and gained the qualifications he needed to set up as a physician recognised by the General Medical Council (GMC), and became a full member of the Royal College of Physicians in 1922 (Kahr, 1996). He decided to specialise in paediatrics.

In 1923 Winnicott took on an appointment as a house physician for children at the Paddington Green Children's Hospital, where he worked for the ensuing forty years. At this clinic, where he saw countless babies and families, he applied his evolving psychoanalytic ideas and put them into practice. He referred to this work as his "psychiatric snack bar", because he found that often it was not possible to offer a full analytic treatment when it was indicated, so, instead, he found that the minimal intervention offered on the basis of psychoanalytic knowledge could very often contribute to a significant improvement in the patient.

There were two other significant events that occurred in 1923. He married Alice Buxton, who was a potter, and he started analysis with James Strachey, who had just returned from a personal analysis in Vienna with Sigmund Freud. By 1926 the Institute of Psychoanalysis established the first psychoanalytic training in the UK. This happened to be the year that Melanie Klein arrived to live in London from Berlin. Winnicott was registered as one of the first candidates in 1927, although he did not begin his training until 1929. He qualified as an adult analyst in 1934 and became the first qualified male child psychoanalyst in 1934.

Three phases of major theoretical achievements

Between 1935 and 1971 the evolution of Winnicott's thought brought about significant elaborations: the environment-individual set-up; transitional phenomena; the use of an object (Abram, 2008). Following qualification as an analyst, Winnicott's working week straddled work as a children's physician and work as an analyst with children and adults in private practice. Although he claimed that he was only able to see babies as human beings as a result of his first five years in analysis, there is no doubt that his continuous work with babies, children, and their families offered him a multitude of insights into the meaning of being a member of a family.

His analysis with James Strachey terminated in 1933, and approximately two years later he started a new analysis with Joan Riviere, one of Melanie Klein's staunch supporters at the time, which was to last for five years. During this time he was also consulting Mrs. Klein for his child cases. Soon, as we can see in his early papers during this period, a certain divergence emerged between his perspective and that of both Riviere and Klein. Winnicott increasingly recognised that the mother's role was of paramount importance to the nascent psyche in a way that he felt Klein did not and could not acknowledge. This point has been emphasised and is at the heart of the differences between Klein and Winnicott (see Abram and Hinshelwood, 2018). But in his later years Winnicott asked the legitimate question: "How to get back to the environment without losing all that was gained by studying the inner factors?" (Winnicott [1967] 1989, p. 577).

This question pervades the work of psychoanalysis and continues to be a highly debated and thought about question. How does it affect technique, for example? How does it affect an understanding of the transference?

The second and third phases of Winnicott's work, which featured transitional phenomena and the use of an object, come directly out of the notion of the environment-individual set-up, as will become clear in the ensuing chapters, and it is my view that while Winnicott knew that he was on to something important in his elaborations, I am not so sure he realised fully that what he was leading to was much more than an elaboration. I suspect this is the same for Bion and was perhaps why he had to move to California from London. We shall see throughout our dialogues. But perhaps the scientific revolutions that both men were evolving could still be seen as unexpected creative bombshells. This may mean that their work is closer than expected given their very different original "stables"; that is, Winnicott was analysed by James Strachey and Bion by Melanie Klein.

CHAPTER FOUR

Psychodynamics and the psychosocial

R.D. Hinshelwood

Group dynamics, 1941–1953

Although Bion was deeply interested in the earliest and most primitive of processes, he never trained as a child analyst. His entry to psychoanalysis was via group dynamics.

In his medical training he had been deeply impressed by one of his teachers at medical school, Wilfred Trotter: "Trotter…listened with unassumed interest as if the patient's contributions flowed from the fount of knowledge itself. It took me years of experience before I learned that this was in fact the case" (Bion, 1985, p 38). In addition, he had developed a profound disdain for the class-based authoritarianism of the British Army, and by the Second World War he was experimenting with different forms of authority which entailed a more collaborative, joint responsibility. His eventual psychotherapy training at the Tavistock Clinic in the 1930s added little to his approach, and it was only when he went into military psychiatry in 1941, with John Rickman as his mentor, that he could begin to fully develop his potential. Rickman encouraged Bion to think about the patient in the context of the ward as a social setting. They formulated their work in terms of what Kurt Lewin called "group dynamics": the individual adopts a role shaped by the social pressures of the group itself (Hinshelwood, 2018).

 DOI: 10.4324/9781003382409-7

Following the war, and during his second analysis with Melanie Klein (1945–1953), Bion journeyed from group dynamics to the psychoanalytic perspective on the individual. In fact, Bion did not abandon his psychosocial point of view, though he had to modify it, influenced by the ideas he gained from his training between 1945 and 1950.

What impressed him in Trotter (as indicated in the quote above) paralleled Klein's approach at this time, as she described herself in her 1936 lectures on technique (recently published):

> If we are not bent on labelling our patients as such and such a type, or wondering prematurely about the structure of the case, if we are not guided in our approach to him by any preconceived plan – trying to evoke such and such response from him – then, and only then, are we ready to learn step by step everything about the patient from himself
> (Steiner, 2017, pp. 29–30).

This kind of openness to the patient as the "fount of knowledge" was a strand of Bion's approach when confronted by patients who violently assaulted the analyst's mind a la the patient in "On hallucinations" (see Part I, dialogue).

From group dynamics to psychoanalysis

From 1948, psychoanalytic concepts reshaped Bion's group experience. Here, for instance, is his attempt to understand the unconscious in terms of group behaviour. He gives a bit of process from a group session and his reaction to it:

MRS. X: I had a nasty turn last week. I was standing in a queue waiting for my turn to go to the cinema when I felt ever so queer. Really, I thought I should faint or something.

MRS. Y: You're lucky to have been going to a cinema. If I thought I could go to a cinema I should feel I had nothing to complain of at all.

MRS. Z: I know what Mrs. X means. I feel just like that myself, only I should have had to leave the queue.

MR. A: Have you tried stooping down? That makes the blood come back to your head. I expect you were feeling faint.

MRS. X: It's not really faint.

MRS. Y: I always find it does a lot of good to try exercises. I don't know if that's what Mr. A means.

MRS. Z: I think you have to use your will-power. That's what worries me – I haven't got any.

MR. B: I had something similar happen to me last week, only I wasn't even standing in a queue. I was just sitting at home quietly when…

MR. C: You were lucky to be sitting at home quietly. If I was able to do that I shouldn't consider I had anything to grumble about.

MRS. Z: I can sit at home quietly all right, but it's never being able to get out anywhere that bothers me. If you can't sit at home, why don't you go to a cinema or something? (Bion, 1948c, pp. 138–139).

This group of patients is in apparently friendly dialogue, yet no one actually connected with anyone else, and

> after listening for some time to this sort of talk, it becomes clear to me that anybody in this group who suffers from a neurotic complaint is going to be advised to do something which the speaker knows from his own experience to be absolutely futile…there is no hope whatever of expecting co-operation from this group.
>
> (Bion, 1948b, p. 139)

The group behaviour lacked focus and seemed futile. No one really collaborated over anyone else's problem, yet Bion was interested that this was a culture that seemed to be supported by everyone in the group. He reflected: "From the way in which the group is going on its motto might be: 'Vendors of quack nostrums unite'" (Bion, 1948b, p. 140). Thus, surprising him, the group's disharmony really displayed itself. They were all co-operative in this un-co-operativeness. This unity was not owned, *consciously*: "I realise that I am expressing my feeling, not of the group's disharmony, but of its unity… The idea that neurotics cannot co-operate has to be modified" (Bion, 1948b, p. 140).

Bion found a psychoanalytic explanation in terms of an unconscious co-operation:

> Some contributions [a member] is prepared to make as coming unmistakably from himself, but there are others which he would wish to make anonymously. If the group can provide means by which contributions can be made anonymously, then the foundations are laid for a successful system of evasion and denial… it was possible because the hostility of the individuals was being contributed to the

> group anonymously that each member could quite sincerely deny that he felt hostile.
>
> (Bion, 1948b, p. 138)

They pooled their unwanted and unacceptable part in a "group mentality". It is clearly a version of the psychoanalytic unconscious in the group. He described, as is well known, three forms of this group mentality, each focused on a basic assumption – dependency, pairing, and fight-flight. He believed these assumptions were innate "valences".

Later, he gave up this psycho-social point of view, stating in a paper for a special issue of the *International Journal of Psychoanalysis* for Klein's seventieth birthday in 1952:

> The understanding of the emotional life of the group, which is a function of the basic assumptions, is only comprehensible in terms of psychotic mechanisms. For this reason advances in the study of the group are dependent upon the development and implications of Melanie Klein's theories of internal objects, projective identification, and failure in symbol formation and their application in the group situation.
>
> (Bion, 1952, p. 247)

At this point, his commitment to Klein's schizoid mechanisms is clear.

Bion's founding commitment to an intuitive listening connected with his training supervisor, Paula Heimann, who gave her seminal paper on countertransference in 1949 (published in 1950). Bion's approach, based in Lewin's social field theory, pointed the analyst towards an introspective grasp of his role based on his feelings in the group, including the analytic group of two. Bion then wrote: "I do not feel quite as happy about postulating a transference situation as I do about postulating a countertransference" (Bion, 1948b, p. 65). He was indicating that his journey in which intuition is an introspective form of listening was continuing.

Conceptualising the roles seen in social field theory can be compared with the personification of objects (or toys) emphasised in Klein's play technique (Klein, 1929). A theory concerning the interaction between objects felt as inside and those seen as outside committed him to a Kleinian perspective until the end of his life, and is evidenced by the characters in his trilogy of novels (Bion, 1975, 1977, 1979).

The psychosis papers of the 1950s

He joined other Kleinians to explore these ideas regarding the treatment of patients in acute psychotic states. The hope and expectation was that these so-called primitive mechanisms would unlock the secret of working with schizophrenic patients, which Freud had not found. The exchanges in these treatments were intense, having a direct and violent impact on the analyst, and Bion regarded them as instances of projective identification.

During the 1950s Bion conformed to these basic Kleinian tenets, and especially to the intensity of the direct exchanges and impact one person makes on others. From 1956 onwards, Bion began to formulate, perhaps more clearly than his Kleinian co-workers, the implications of these direct exchanges as forms of containment: "Melanie Klein has described how this mechanism produces problems for the patient by engendering fear of the analyst who now is a container of a bad part of himself" (Bion, 1958, p. 342). He then focused on a receptivity to intrusions of the bits and pieces of a rejected self. This receptivity he eventually called "reverie".

He and several colleagues were beginning to describe a step forwards in describing projective identification and receiving it as a form of communication – not the communication of information, but the unsymbolised transfer of direct experiences. It may have been Heimann's influence that helped Bion postulate this communicative form, in contrast to the more psychotic, evacuative form of projective identification. Here is Bion's vivid formulation:

> When the patient strove to rid himself of fears of death which were felt to be too powerful for his personality to contain he split off his fears and put them into me, the idea apparently being that if they were allowed to repose there long enough they would undergo modification by my psyche and could then be safely reintrojected.
>
> (Bion, 1959, p 147)

Hanna Segal strongly agreed with this model of the container-contained, and later emphasised the re-introjection as the acquisition by the patient of the capacity to modify his own fears for himself. Bion had implied that such a containing process does not always run smoothly or successfully, and Segal succinctly said: "A great deal can go wrong in the projection. The relation between the container and the contained may be felt as mutually destructive or mutually emptying" (Segal, 1978, p 317).

At the time of writing his paper "Attacks on linking", in 1957 (published 1959), the book *Envy and Gratitude* had been published by

Klein amid controversy. The "attacks" in the title of the paper refer to an examination of the envy aroused by containers, an envy which is at the root of the problems that Segal summarised. However, the paper diverted towards the description of containing as the source of envy: the object is envied because it establishes the subject as so dependent and inadequate in comparison.

Bion's model of container-contained had a great future ahead as a paradigm for therapeutic work in psychoanalysis until the present day. Klein died shortly after, in 1960, and Bion seemed to feel released to begin what he intended to be a specifically Kleinian metapsychology (see Chapter 6). His success in the 1950s in evolving the model of container-contained owed a good deal to his psychosocial work with groups, and a seed can perhaps be seen in that formulation of group mentality whereby the group contains the repudiated and anonymised parts of the individuals.

Summary

Much of this part is taken up with the nature of interpretation and the view, following classical Freudian psychoanalysis, that understanding the intolerable involves repeating a past trauma in the present. The alternative view is that not understanding, or not expressing understanding, is a denial in the present of something intolerable that prevails in the unconscious.

Moreover, the intolerable is conceived differently by each author. For Bion it is the experience of an "other" that destroys the self so that the sense of being or of having an ego-boundary with the rest of the world disintegrates. However, this initial sense of a self, or of an ego, does not exist from the outset for Winnicott, for whom an unintegrated collection of experiences come to be established and integrated into a self. This collection of ego functions, which for Bion is fragilely integrated, includes a significant function – that of knowing. Bion emphasised this in his period where he studied the development of knowing, but it connected with Klein's early work on the ability of children to learn when learning may come close to an intolerable knowledge, such as of parental intercourse (primal scene) and the Oedipal situation.

It is the knowledge inherent in an interpretation which is therapeutic, bringing the intolerable into a tolerable form. While this is perhaps true for both Winnicott and Bion, there is still a difference. For Bion this process of knowing the intolerable enhances and adds to the strength of the ego, while Winnicott emphasises the facilitation of awareness comes from the mother's holding, which includes the capacity to receive intolerable affective states that the infant is not able to tolerate. This particular aspect of holding resonates with Bion's container-contained model. Bion nevertheless acknowledged that the strength the other can become, through internalisation, an internal strength for the ego.

Prior to qualifying as psychoanalysts, Bion and Winnicott had significantly different experiences, as different as those of a paediatrician and a group therapist. Nevertheless, both shared an interest in the social context of the patient – Winnicott in the family in the past, and Bion in a social group in the present. Both were therefore intent, as Winnicott said, to return to the social environment while retaining the psychoanalytic knowledge of the unconscious and the inner world, as Bion would call it. They achieved this in different ways; Winnicott postulated a third area – transitional phenomena: neither me nor not-me. Bion, consistent with Klein, postulated an inner world of dreamlike activity, the objects of which could be exchanged or could distort.

Table 2 Early foundations

Winnicott	*Bion*
1. He qualified as both a child analyst as well as an adult analyst	1. He firstly studied the earliest and most primitive processes in group dynamics
2. The patient is seen as a member of a family	2. The patient is seen in a social context
3. The crucial setting is the environment-individual setup	3. The patient is in a role shaped by the social pressures of a group
4. Winnicott stressed the environment as well as the study of inner factors	4. Bion evolved his basic assumptions of groups as collaborative psychotic mechanisms
5. He postulated transitional phenomena and the use of an object	5. The perception of objects interacts with actual external objects
6. There are developmental stages in the use of an object	6. The external object is used partly as a container to receive projective identifications
7. It is believed that Klein could not acknowledge the mother's role in development	7. Projective identification has a direct and violent impact on the maternal container
	8. Bion was less to define the transference than he was the countertransference
	9. Crucial to the container-contained model are the attacks on that containing link

Dialogue

Jan Abram: Bion's revelation that it took him years to recognise the value of Trotter's approach to his patients' contributions as containing the "fount of knowledge itself" is completely in line with Winnicott's writing, "The principle is that it is the patient and only the patient who has the answers" (Winnicott, 1969a). This sentence of Winnicott's, however, is related to his view about the technique of interpretation, and carried an indirect criticism of the "making of interpretations" rather than of interpretations per se. He wrote, "I think I interpret mainly to let the patient know the limits of my understanding". Winnicott, in his 1969 paper, implied a criticism of "over-interpretation" in any given analysis. He reflects on "how much deep change" he had prevented in the past by his personal need to interpret – especially for patients in a "certain classification category" – referring to borderline patients. I have always understood that Winnicott was really referring to what he perceived as a propensity in Kleinian technique to over-interpret. There has been much discussion in the British Psychoanalytical Society over the different theoretical orientations, where the Independents and Contemporary Freudians tend to offer less interpretations than the Kleinians seem to. So, I must admit to feeling surprised when, at the beginning of this chapter, you make the case that Bion, following Klein, advocated an openness to the patient as the "fount of knowledge". Could you elaborate on how this is illustrated in Bion's essay "On hallucination"? I am interested in how you will illustrate this because I think the notion of "openness" and of recognising the patient's contribution appear to be compatible, especially between Bion and Winnicott, but are actually quite different. For example, how does the analyst convey to the patient that their contribution (the patient's) carries a knowledge about themselves? We could ask the same question of Winnicott's sentence. How does the analyst convey to the patient that they are the one with the answers?

Robert D. Hinshelwood: Yes, I guess there is an age-old dispute which started with Anna Freud's (1927) claim that interpretation of children was never going to be effective. And Klein (1932) showed with evidence that the impact of interpreting the unconscious was effective even in the youngest. My guess is that Winnicott would have initially agreed with Klein. As far as Bion was concerned, I think the debate evolved to something more complex. From early in his work, and in his pre-psychoanalytic days, he clearly expected a joint responsibility between patients and therapist. For instance, in his 1942 experiment in wartime, he ended one daily parade of the men with this comment:

> The problem, I said, appeared to be one that not only concerned the training wing, or even the Army alone… . I suggested that they should study it and come forward with fresh proposals when they felt they were beginning to see daylight.
>
> (Bion, 1961, p. 19)

Much later, James Gooch recalled from his analysis with Bion in the 1970s that Bion would say something like, "Well, this or that that you said suggests that it's correct but we'll have to wait to know till you can feel it" (Culbert-Koehn, 2011, p. 81). I think it is quite true that in 1956, when he presented his paper "On hallucination" (published 1958), he was working very differently and was keen to demonstrate the effectiveness of Klein's schizoid mechanisms.

I think this demonstrates some difficulties we have. First, that Bion radically changed his thinking and practice at different times, though this is an instance when he reverted later to an earlier form of interpretation which remains therefore more characteristic. Secondly, we do have to confront impressions handed down through the generations that one school of analysts has of another school.

But there is a further issue that I think Bion gradually made clear. That is, we are working together with the conscious patient to understand their unconscious. By definition, the patient cannot consciously speak of his unconscious. Or if he does, it is intellectual sophistication. The patient's unconscious speaks to us in transference enactments and impacts directly and non-symbolically on the analyst.

You touched on an important issue in our discussion of clinical paradigms, and it leads into Bion's notions of containing and catastrophic change. We may be continuing a debate we had previously about Winnicott's fear of interpretations as something that disturbs the necessary experience of omnipotence for the patient. It intrigues me to know what sort of "snacks" (of psychoanalysis) Winnicott offered in his paediatric work, which could have been effective in healing the wound of a premature rupture in primary omnipotence.

The other useful issue, it seems to me, is the one you end on in Chapter 3 – how to get back to the environment. Could Winnicott know the specific environmental mother that the patient had? How can we know her? And what can be done with her?

J.A.: It's helpful to be reminded of the early disagreements that Klein's work with children seemed to instigate in Vienna during the late 1920s and 1930s on technique. Anna Freud's model for child analysis was quite different, as you point out. This was not only related to the issue of technique but also to the different ways in which Anna Freud and Melanie Klein viewed the notion of transference in young children.

I am reminded of a discussion at the beginning of my training, in the early 1980s, with a colleague of mine who was training to be a child analyst at the Tavistock Clinic. We were sharing our ideas about this very topic and she gave me an example of giving an interpretation to a young child of about five years of age. After her interpretation, the young child looked up at her and asked, "How did you know that?" For my colleague this was evidence indeed that the interpretation had worked. At the time I felt slightly stunned, but I've never forgotten that her example of giving a "deep" interpretation from her understanding of the child's unconscious, which was being illustrated through the child's play, was what worked. At one level it seemed convincing, but much later I started to reflect on the child's question. Perhaps, indeed, the child did feel understood at that moment. On the other hand, it occurred to me that the child is likely to have felt that the therapist (my colleague) "knew" something that they did not. Rather like a parent or a GP telling a young child why they have a tummy ache. When any one of us is disconcerted and afraid of what is happening to us psychologically and/or somatically, actually at any age, we are very relieved to find a person who "knows" and understands our position. So when Winnicott writes that "interpretation outside the ripeness of time amounts to indoctrination", he is referring to one of the major pitfalls in psychoanalytic practice whereby an interpretation that bypasses the patient's preconscious risks being a kind of indoctrination (Winnicott, 1969a). I don't think Kleinians are the only analysts who risk this, but I do think that if there is an overemphasis on making the "correct interpretation", then the risk of indoctrination is higher.

It is also striking that you say Bion gradually got something clear when he recognised the issue of the manifestation of the unconscious through transference enactments. But, as I'm sure you know, from the beginning of technique in Classical Freudian analysis, following Anna Freud and her colleagues, the analyst makes an interpretation that they feel the patient is able to tolerate because it is not going straight to the unconscious but rather the conscious/pre-conscious layer of the patient's awareness. The patient may or may not "enact" or indeed "act out", but Classical analysts listen to the derivatives of the unconscious and decide on how to "pitch" the interpretation. This approach stems from an awareness that interpretations can be traumatising. Winnicott, according to some of his patients, worked along these lines. We looked at this in Part V of our first book, and in Chapter 10, "Holding and the mutative interpretation", I argued that interpretations would mean nothing to the patient unless they were given in a holding environment. I'll take this point up again in Part III of this book. But it brings me to the question of the environment mother, and your questions: How can we know her and what can be done with her? The short answer to these questions lies in the nature of the evolving transference-countertransference matrix. Winnicott is not alone in thinking that while it will never be possible to know the patient's real mother, it is possible to have an experience of the *patient's version* of their mother through what is mobilised due to the analysing situation. As I pointed out in the IPA webinar on holding and containing on 11 April 2021, when we were examining aspects of the infantile in the work of Winnicott and Bion, the infantile, for Winnicott, constitutes the multitude of infantile experiences that the newborn has gradually constructed in relation to the psychic environment.

I went on to propose the notion of an intrapsychic clinical infant, following Daniel Stern's use of this term: "Who will come to light in the patient exclusively through the transference-countertransference" (Abram, 2021).

I will finish with another point that is pertinent to the differences between how both of our authors worked and their different clinical paradigms and techniques. Winnicott made very clear that if the patient could not "do analysis", then the analyst has to do "something else" (Winnicott, 1960). This brings up another controversy about how analysts work with psychotic (and borderline) patients. For Winnicott it was necessary to wait until the patient could "play" in the psychoanalytic sense. I know there were many Kleinians during a particular phase in the history of psychoanalysis who worked with psychotic patients and had evidence it worked. In reference to our IPA webinar again, you presented Bion's clinical material (from his paper on the psychotic and non-psychotic parts of the personality that underpins his paper "On Hallucination"), and I responded to it by citing Winnicott's letter to Bion illustrating how differently he would have worked with the patient. To my mind, what Winnicott would have offered relates to the reality principle. In reference to your remark that Bion had a radical change in his work from the 1960s on, I wonder if, looking back, he would have worked more along the lines that Winnicott was suggesting in 1958.

R.D.H.: I think you put a finger on the important question – how to know if one's interpretation is correct. As you know, there is a bit of literature about this which fades off into philosophy and epistemology. Grunbaum (1984) took Freud at his word when Freud talked of the interpretation "tallying" with something in the patient (Freud, 1917), and I did take this up in my book on research (Hinshelwood, 2013). It is only the patient who can tell if an interpretation is the "right" one. I am sure we would agree. But Freud knew it was not a conscious agreement which mattered, but rather a change in the transference enactments that give the indication. You may know Klein's case of Rita (aged four), so persecuted by strangers and the analyst in particular that she would not relate to the analyst at all. Klein found it necessary for the older (adolescent) sister to remain in the room during the session. After an interpretation by Klein of the little girl's hateful phantasies of her mother having a new baby, the girl turned to the analyst and played with her for the first time. This is quite different from a conscious agreement.

I am interested that Winnicott wanted to "pitch" his interpretations, and that they could only be made in a safe holding situation. It makes it sound like an avoidance of something. You would call it trauma, but I think Kleinians would say that Winnicott's pitching is to avoid something persecuting, something intolerable that is to be defended against. Well, in ordinary conversation that is what one does. But in a psychoanalysis, surely the need is to face the intolerable in some way. Is it that only being nice counts? It is not enough to play safe. If the analyst is seen as persecuting, then that is the construction of the patient – and then a further interpretation. Patients feel faced with the intolerable, and that feels like an object that is intent on persecuting or traumatising them. That is transference, and it is very important what you say about the "patient's version". The mother is not seen as she actually is, any more than the analyst is. You are conveying now that it is not the actual mother that is important ! Isn't it true that we all explore the patient's version, all the time? Surely we agree on this. As Kant conveyed, we only see the appearances that we make of reality. Where do our experiences come from? As you say, "The newborn has gradually constructed [its version of mother] in relation to the psychic environment". I am sure we are in absolute agreement.

How does the infant construct? That is the work of analysis. On what principles and dimensions and categories and emotional convictions (and so on)? I guess you would say, and I would agree, that this is not neglecting the actual environment, only recognising the infant's limited reality principle at the beginning. We have to be interested in that construction process.

Going back to the question of avoiding the persecuting experiences in the analytic session, how does Winnicott think this can be tackled if he wants to try to avoid the experience in the analysis?

Again, I think if we agree that facing the worst is the essence of the analytic process, then how do we do it? For Bion, it is an issue of containing. That is, of converting the unsymbolised enactment into a verbally contained set of comprehensions. I am concerned that we could come away with the idea that Winnicott thinks we face the unfaceable by making it comfortable and safe. In effect, that would seem to be a bit like a collusion to deny the worst.

Perhaps this is one critical difference between holding and containing. In containing, the relation with the analyst is one in which, together, the worst can be faced for what it is and can be made more manageable by containing it in a represented, symbolic, verbal form. In holding, perhaps, there is a necessary provision of comfort. For Bion there is love, there is hate, but there is a third thing. That is the capacity to represent and to know, in that specifically human way, the internal representation which Freud learned from his philosophy teacher Franz Brentano and which led to his model of thing-presentation plus word-presentation resulting in the conscious "object-presentation" (see Strachey, 1975).

Thus, there is really a considerable amount of agreement, I think, about the act of interpreting, but the significant divergence is in Bion's model of an impulse to know alongside the loving and hating. This impulse to know is an added dimension to interpretation. The encouragement of the patient to know the worst rubs off on them as an identification with an ego of superior strength (although one which is often resented as such). This encouragement to face the worst together is not lacking in persecution. It creates an important situation whereby the patient needs the analyst while also hating them as a persecutor (because they have superior ego-strength). Such a situation of ambivalence and concern constitutes the depressive position in Klein's terms.

One concern, to my mind, would be the possibility that Winnicott pitched things so carefully and was so concerned about the comfort and safety of holding that he missed the true prevalence and significance of the intolerable (and thus the paranoid-schizoid position). Of course, there is a risk that to lead the patient into his own intolerable sense of persecution will destroy the analysis (if not the patient), and care needs to be taken to pace this correctly. Patients who are amenable to analytic treatments will have some part of their ego that can appreciate the analyst's willingness to face the worst with them. Freud himself pointed to this robust element of the patient's ego when he talked of quite psychotic patients thus:

> One learns from patients after their recovery that at the time in some corner of their mind (as they put it) there was a normal person hidden, who, like a detached spectator, watched the hubbub of illness go past him.
>
> (Freud, 1938, p. 202)

And it is necessary to have confidence that such a willingness and capacity exists in one's patient without having to avoid the persecution.

You ask, finally, if Bion was aware of Winnicott's 1958 description of his practice. Bion did his best not to acknowledge Winnicott in any way. But it seems to me that quite frequently Bion did follow up an idea of Winnicott's, without acknowledgement, and re-expressed it in Kleinian terms. The development of containing as a Kleinian version of holding may have been a case in point.

J.A.: We are finding ourselves discussing difference in technique, which inevitably relate to different ways of interpreting. And yet, when we start to home in on the details, we find there is agreement about the nuances of interpretation, and as you remind us, this is not new in psychoanalysis: there is a huge literature on the topic. But to examine Winnicott's approach from Bion's is our main aim here. In Part V of our book on Klein and Winnicott we examined practice and theory, and I remember it being one of the most difficult dialogues, and we agreed to differ ultimately, but I feel the same misunderstandings are coming up again, although Bion's change in his late work may well have departed from the Kleinian technique we know today. Most London Kleinians reject Bion's late work, don't they?

I think – and it seems you think too – that Bion was very influenced by Winnicott but did not refer to his work or allow himself to be influenced by his work while he, Bion, was developing his way of working that differed from his early work. You gave me the impression that Bion was working quite differently at the end of his clinical practice in comparison with his clinical work as seen in the papers in *Second Thoughts* (Bion, 1957, 1958).

I do remember you mentioning how Klein allowed Rita's sister to stay in the room until she was ready to be with Klein on her own, and I also remember saying I thought this was a good example of "doing something else" rather than staying with the "pure technique" of analysis. From Winnicott's point of view, I think Mrs. Klein showed flexibility about the setting in order to build up a sense of trust in her little patient. Perhaps it could be seen as a normal response that Rita was wary of strangers and might well be to do with something that had happened to her rather than her inhibitions being *only* because of her internal persecutors. I think this could be a good example of our different approaches. I tend to see inhibition in the patient as a combination of what happened and what they imagine happened. The process of analysis teases out differences, even though we can never be definitively sure about fantasies and/or reality. It's always an admixture.

I do feel you misunderstand the notion of "pitching" an interpretation as avoidant on Winnicott's part. In fact, what I pointed out was that Winnicott was following a Classical Freudian way of working whereby the analyst attempts an interpretation that they feel the patient can accept and, more importantly, make use of. Moreover, I don't think this is intended as "being nice" but rather as doing what Klein did with Rita – building up a sense of trust. It takes a very long time for a patient to develop a capacity to really examine the most unpleasant and disturbing aspects of the personality, such as hate and death wishes.

My emphasis on appreciating that the transference is always a "version" of the patient's mother/environment is because, so often, it seems there is a misunderstanding of Winnicott's emphasis on early psychic development as "actual". You say we're in "absolute agreement" about this, and yet the question we're left with concerns how we understand the different versions of the patient, because there are always going to be elements of the real mother/environment. But it is surely true that this can never be totally verified.

The question of how the infant is constructed relates to how the adult patient on the couch constructs their own infantile experiences, which will involve the unconscious, preconscious, and conscious mind. You're right that I would agree that we cannot totally neglect the actual environment in this process. But when you say that this is based on the recognition that the infant's reality principle is limited at the beginning, I do not agree with you. I would say, following Winnicott, that the infant has no idea – yet – what the reality principle means. The reality principle evolves because of the mother's mediation of the infant's demands and needs from the very beginning. What's more, without a facilitating environment, the awareness of the reality principle is impossible to reach. That's why the psychotic is not in a position to make "use of the object" and play, in Winnicott's language.

Your question regarding the avoidance of persecuting experiences is a crucial one. Winnicott, in my reading of his work, does not advocate avoidance at any point in his work. What he proposes is that if the patient is profoundly traumatised from birth, then it will make an enormous difference as to whether they have the capacity to make use of the analytic setting.

This "fact" of early trauma, then, brings us to the issue that inevitably relates to how to work with borderline/psychotic patients. Do we adjust analytic technique depending on the patient's pathology. For Winnicott, it is absolutely necessary to adapt to the patient's psychohistory, but this does not mean avoiding what the patient will, in time, have to recognise in themselves.

It reminds me of a patient in analysis for ten years who took a good seven years of five weekly sessions before she could truly feel and acknowledge that her real mother was not a witch who was out to kill her. You, or your colleagues, might say that she would have got to this quicker with a Kleinian analyst. That is perhaps something that is complex to prove.

The issue of which approach is right or wrong is manifestly overdetermined. We both know from the analyses we have undergone that the approach was, presumably, good. It made us the analysts we have become and are still becoming. We also know of many analysts who were unhappy with the kind of analysis they had. Many Kleinian analysts have moved to Freudians and/or Independents because they felt persecuted by too many interpretations, and many analysts who were analysed by Independents or Contemporary Freudians moved to a Kleinian because they felt that something had been ignored or possibly avoided. But it's also true that many analysts select an analyst on the basis of personality and feel it appropriate to have a second analysis. The first analysis cannot always reach certain aspects of the personality; perhaps especially in a training analysis. There's no such thing as an ideal analysis, or is there? What is the evidence for and indeed meaning of a successful analysis?

I don't fully agree with the way you are describing the differences between holding and containing, and I feel we're moving to the third part of this book. Like many of our exchanges, it does feel crucial to start bringing in some clinical examples to highlight our points. But before we do, I want to return to something else you discuss in Chapter 4 on psychodynamics and the psychosocial. The equivalent study for Winnicott is to be seen in his paediatric practice and his therapeutic consultations, in which can be seen the examples of "snack bar therapy" (Winnicott, 1971c). In this way, both men were elaborating on the application of psychoanalysis – Bion to groups and Winnicott to families. Much more has been explored in these areas which could be referred to as psychosocial by many other authors.

How striking that Paula Heimann was Bion's supervisor and that he said he was more interested in the countertransference than in the transference. This must have brought him into some conflict with Klein I would have thought, as she did not accept this concept and indeed tried to stop Paula Heimann giving her paper at the IPA conference in 1949. This was the very moment that Heimann left the Klein group, was it not? It made me wonder how Bion managed this.

I'm sure we'll continue to explore these points as we move on to the next parts, but it seems to me that we're ready to embark on Part III now.

R.D.H.: There are so many points to make in response to your last contribution, but many may come later. I do feel that there is a bit of repetition in the sense that we are making differences out of what are in fact similarities. I don't entirely go along with the persistence of Winnicottians in claiming Klein neglected the external environment. That was why I picked up on your point about the "constructed mother" that the infant has. On what principles or grounds does the infant make his constructions? We can't say that the infant is both totally formed by the environment and at the same time that they contributes his own construction of it. So I think we are in complete agreement when you say that "we can never be definitively sure about fantasies and/or reality. It's always an admixture". The issue is whether we are interested in the fantasies the infant has about his reality, or simply in the reality of the environment mother. It is as if there is a necessity to polarise Winnicottians and Kleinians in this respect.

Can I put it as succinctly as possible? When an infant is overwhelmed by some experience, he feels, well...overwhelmed. It threatens something so awful that it is beyond imagining and coping. Kleinians would call it persecution – the feeling of being destroyed by the experience. Winnicottians would call it trauma. I wonder if we could agree to equate the feeling of being persecuted to the point of one's being going out of existence (Klein) with the feeling of being so traumatised one's continuity of being is lost (Winnicott). For me, a Kleinian, they are the same. Are they different for a Winnicottian? My sense is that this is just the kind of thing that Klein and Winnicott were in parallel on and probably discussing together between the 1920s and 1940s. It was only after 1950, as you say, that things turned sour and each had to prove the other wrong. My concern is that we must not simply rehearse the misunderstandings of their later non-collaboration but should also remember their earlier collaboration.

Our aim here is to move on from this and to try to focus more specifically on the comparisons of Bion's specific contribution.

In respect of the last point, I want to take up your point about "different ways of interpreting". Moving more explicitly to Bion's development of Klein, he makes it clear it that is not just a different way of interpreting but that there are different aims in making an interpretation. It may be that Winnicott was classical in seeing interpretation as making conscious (in some carefully graduated way) what is unconscious in the patient. Bion, however, saw this differently, and it is implied in Klein, certainly from around the early 1930s. It is not about the contents of the mind and the unconscious, but about the ability of the mind to function as a mind at all. As Bion put it:

> The non-psychotic personality was concerned with a neurotic problem, that is to say a problem that centred on the resolution of a conflict of ideas and emotions to which the operation of the ego had given rise. But the psychotic personality was concerned with the problem of repair of the ego.
>
> (Bion, 1957, p. 272)

It may well be the case that Winnicott interprets at that level of unconscious conflict, but the sense of his meaning of trauma is much more akin to Klein's, and Bion's view of a serious threat and damage to the ego itself and not simply conflict. As for Bion, there are these two absolutely clear-cut differences regarding the level of interpretation; it would be interesting to know if Winnicott acknowledged such a difference between conflict anxiety and survival anxiety, or whether it appears to be a false distinction in Winnicott's terms.

The aim of an interpretation for Bion is therefore to deal with the disintegration (I believe Winnicott would call it unintegration) before there can be a real approach to the neurotic conflicts.

Incidentally, you are right that Klein did modify classical technique in her work in the early 1920s – that is, if we assume there was a classical technique then. It has always seemed to me that the strictness of technique was something that evolved, especially in the late 1920s and until the late 1930s. But this is a separate point. And the example of Rita was to show that a "deep" interpretation, even in someone so young (aged four), resulted in a radical, immediate change in the patient's trust and capacity to relate, and that it did not depend on a slow build-up of trust. Understanding had an immediate effect.

J.A.: I feel what I'm trying to do, Bob, is to elaborate rather than repeat. Paradoxically, this means going over the same issues that were fraught in the psyche's past and which remain so in the present. I'd like to pick up on some of the points you make with some further elaboration.

Differences and similarities

There are similarities, I agree, if we are referring to interpretation that aims to assist the patient in feeling what they don't know they are feeling and seeing what they are not yet able to see about themselves and the world around them. We'd both call that the ability to discern self and other, I imagine. However, different approaches will bring about different ways of interpreting. In order to really illuminate the differences, we need to bring in some clinical material, and I hope we will come to this very point in Part III, when we examine Bion's clinical material in his paper on the psychotic and non-psychotic personalities and discuss it in relation to Winnicott's suggestion to Bion about a very different way of interpreting. When we discussed this in the first IPA webinar, the differences in approach were substantial, you'll remember, and I feel it's important to re-examine them and deepen our discussion, which was time limited due to the conditions of the webinar.

Klein's neglect of the external environment

The case of Rita, to my mind, shows that Klein's technique was flexible. But when you say that there was no build-up of trust in her work with her little patient, I find it difficult to agree that it was only understanding that made the difference to Rita's improvement. I think this issue is relevant to Bion's clinical examples too. A normal process of building up trust takes place in every relationship, whether it is analytic or not.

On what principles does the infant make his constructions?

This question you pose is quite crucial to the distinction between the Kleinian and Winnicottian clinical paradigm. I think Winnicott learnt a great deal from being in supervision with Melanie Klein during the 1920s and '30s, but by the late 1930s, and especially during the Controversial Discussions, he was sharpening his ideas and finding himself with a very different perspective on what happened to the infant at the very beginning. This is where the actuality of the mother comes in. She was either able to hold her infant or not. Yes – I'm repeating myself here, but I feel it needs more clarification relative to what you say about the baby being overwhelmed.

For Winnicott – and I think this applies to Bion's container-contained – the baby will only be overwhelmed *if* the mother is not able to hold him, which involves protection from "primitive agonies" and "falling forever".

When you draw a parallel between persecution in Kleinian theory and trauma in Winnicott's, I do see your point of view. But – and this is essential to spell out – trauma is *not* de facto. This is why the concept of the paranoid-schizoid position in Klein's theory is rejected by Winnicott as a universal experience for *all* babies. I outlined in Chapter 4 of our first book that for Winnicott there are two babies: one baby ontologically knows about the holding environment, and the other baby ontologically knows about primitive agonies. And this observation of Winnicott's directly relates to his distinction between conflict anxiety and survival anxiety, as you asked.

So, these are the principles on which the baby makes his constructions, and depending on the early environment they will either become psychotic or neurotic constructs – more or less.

Differentiating between fantasy and reality

The analyst, then, through their transference-countertransference, will become aware of the infantile layers in the adult and start to differentiate between the psychotic and non-psychotic layers. But for Winnicott the psychotic layer does not exist in every patient. That will depend on the early holding environment. I think this relates to Bion's theory of container-contained, although it is different because based on the different paradigms.

Difference between unintegration and disintegration

You say that Bion's aim in interpreting is to deal with the patient's disintegration, and you say in parenthesis that Winnicott would call it unintegration. This is misleading. Unintegration for Winnicott is the state in which the newborn comes into the world. There can be no disintegration until there has been a certain amount of integration. The infant's ability to integrate physiology with psychology can only come about through the mother's mediation, which is all part and parcel of her ability to hold the infant.

I would just like to say one more word on the citation of Bion's. I think Winnicott would agree with the first sentence – that the non-psychotic personality is concerned with resolution of conflict. But when Bion says that the psychotic personality is "concerned with the problem of repair of the ego", I think Winnicott would say that the psychotic personality is concerned with the early deficiency of the psychic environment which had caused early psychic trauma. Therefore, the psychotic's effort to "repair the ego" is a kind of reparation of the deficient mother, who was not able to provide what the early infant needed.

R.D.H.: Only one final point: this is what you refer to as the psychotic functioning. When you say that the baby (or infant in the adult patient) "is concerned with the early deficiency of the psychic environment", it seems unlikely that the baby will have a concept of the psychic environment, but instead will experience it in their own "baby" terms. Where Winnicott and Bion would differ is in the way they perceive the object. For Winnicott it might be an object (mother) which just lets the baby drop, alone and unheld; for Bion (following Klein here) it would be an object (mother) that is seen as malevolent and as having an *intention* to drop and destroy the infant.

I think the Bion view adds two things to Winnicott's. One is that we have to stick with the narratives that a baby might use and experience. And the other is that an object, for Bion's baby, has an intention itself, while for Winnicott the object is not personified with its own purpose.

PART III

THE PRINCIPLE FORMULATIONS

Chapters 5 and 6 outline the key formulations – holding and containing – predicated on Winnicott's investigation of the maternal role and on Bion's several alternative paradigms. These theories are outlined with reference to the basic assumptions of both authors.

DOI: 10.4324/9781003382409-8

CHAPTER FIVE

Holding

Jan Abram

The concept of holding emerged in Winnicott's work in the mid 1950s to identify the myriad functions of the mother's role for her newborn. The theory of holding evolved up until Winnicott's death and has now become one of those concepts that is associated with containing. There is often a misperception that holding is "just holding" and less complex than Bion's theory of container-contained, but holding is one of the key concepts in Winnicott's clinical paradigm as it defines the essential function of the parent-infant relationship.

The holding environment

Winnicott's focus is on the emotional holding-the-baby-in-mind in combination with the physical feeding, bathing, and dressing. The infant, Winnicott says, only understands love that is expressed in human terms "by live, human holding... we are more concerned with the mother *holding* the baby than with the mother *feeding* the baby" (Winnicott, 1955, pp. 147–148). This emphasis is to stress that if the mother is totally engaged through her identification with her baby (primary maternal preoccupation), then feeding will be something that occurs as a consequence of the emotional engagement.

DOI: 10.4324/9781003382409-9

It is because of the holding environment – or through the holding environment – that the infant is facilitated to develop the capacity to integrate experience and develop the sense of "I am *me*" ("Me"). Winnicott suggested that the I AM process is a "raw moment" because the new infant feels infinitely exposed. Therefore, the mother's full identification with her infant is necessary, which means the I AM moment can be endured. This is during the very earliest stages of Absolute Dependence – the holding phase.

By 1960, Winnicott's definitive statement on holding appears in his paper "The theory of the parent-infant relationship". The holding environment necessarily includes the father.

Satisfactory parental care can be classified roughly into three overlapping stages:

> a. Holding
> b. Mother and infant living together. Here the father's function (of dealing with the environment for the mother) is not known.
> c. Father, mother, and infant, all three living together
>
> (Winnicott, 1960, p. 589)

"Living together" refers to the infant's ability to separate "Me" from "Not-me" and to see mother and father as separate, whole people. But this can only occur as a consequence of a successful holding by the parents from the beginning. This leads to an appreciation of reality and to a "three dimensional or space relationship with time gradually added" (Winnicott, 1960, p. 589).

The holding function

The function of holding means that the mother is able to discern her infant's needs rather than impose on the infant what she thinks they need. This ability to recognise the infant as a separate, evolving personality is key to the infant's emotional development of self. Awareness of body as distinct from emotions gradually evolves through sensitive holding. The environment must be reliable, not in a mechanical way but rather with an emphasis on reliability. This relates to the mother's empathy emanating from her deep identification with her infant's sense of helplessness.

The protection from physical and psychological insult takes account of the infant's acute skin sensitivity, visual sensitivity, and sensitivity to gravity, because the infant at the very start is not yet aware of a distinction between self and other.

Good-enough holding at the beginning, carried out by the mother, with the father enabling her total dedication to the infant, will mean that the infant will also be protected from trauma. If the holding environment is not good enough, the infant will suffer a psychic break in the continuity-of-being, a traumatic rupture that could result in psychosis. In fact, for Winnicott the psychotic or borderline patient has indeed suffered early psychic trauma because of the deficiency of holding during the holding phase.

Personalisation

An important aspect of holding is what Winnicott refers to as "handling" – the way the mother handles her infant in the day-to-day details of infant care. Her enjoyment of her infant and her *desire* to handle and hold are an expression of love. This function leads to the psyche-in-dwelling-in-the-soma (Abram, 2007, pp. 263–274), which depicts a process of personalisation. This means that the infant comes to feel, because of loving handling, that their body is themselves and that the sense of self is centred in the body.

The term "personalisation" is used to accentuate the opposite of depersonalisation – the condition in which the individual experiences a mind-body split and does not feel integrated with their body: "Being loved at the beginning means being accepted…the child has a blueprint for normality which is largely a matter of the shape and functioning of their body" (Winnicott, 1971, p. 264). In his very late work, Winnicott stressed "acceptance" as a sign of being loved and how this is shown in the physical care of the infant, which starts long before the actual birth experience.

> The beginning of that part of the baby's development which I am calling personalisation, or which can be described as an indwelling of the psyche in the soma, is to be found in the mother's ability to join up her emotional involvement, which originally is physical and psychological.
> (Winnicott, 1971, p. 264)

In the analytic situation, it is the analyst's attention – in combination with the physicality of the environment, the couch, the warmth, the aesthetics of the room – that mirrors the mother's actual body and her psychic primary maternal preoccupation.

Therapeutic management

The holding environment is a form of management, Winnicott wrote, for the child and adolescent whose symptoms are antisocial. The staff working in children's residential therapeutic communities also required a specialised form of holding (see Britton and Winnicott, 1947).

The analyst's attention, along with and including interpretative work, constitutes the holding environment of any given psychoanalytic treatment. Only from the fact of holding can a potential space be realised and a sense of self start to flourish.

CHAPTER SIX

Transformations

R.D. Hinshelwood

Developed in the 1950s, Bion's (1959) model of container-contained had a great future ahead as a paradigm for therapeutic work in psychoanalysis until the present day. Klein died shortly after its publication, in 1960, and Bion seemed to feel released to begin what was intended to be a specifically Kleinian metapsychology.

After these careful explorations of clinical practice, by the 1960s Bion had amassed sufficient experience to formulate abstractions and theories. He had become a member of the British Psychoanalytical Society during the long aftermath of the Controversial Discussions, and may have been deeply affected by both the lingering animosity to Klein and the competitive certainties of differing psychoanalytic schools.

Briefly from the 1950s

Bion and others were using the idea of relationships in which fragmented bits of experience and ego are projected into the analyst – a process called projective identification. By 1955, they were beginning to think that projective identification might take another form, one with the aim of a kind of communication. Bion's 1959 paper formulated this, and its aim is very clear:

DOI: 10.4324/9781003382409-10

> When the patient strove to rid himself of fears of death which were felt to be too powerful for his personality to contain he split off his fears and put them into me, the idea apparently being that if they were allowed to repose there long enough they would undergo modification by my psyche and could then be safely reintrojected.
>
> (Bion, 1959, p. 312)

He thought this was a direct, non-symbolic form of communication typical of early infancy:

> From the infant's point of view she should have taken into her, and thus experienced, the fear that the child was dying. It was this fear that the child could not contain. He strove to split it off together with the part of the personality in which it lay and project it into the mother. An understanding mother is able to experience the feeling of dread that this baby was striving to deal with by projective identification and yet retain a balanced outlook.
>
> (Bion, 1959, pp. 312–313)

This clearly conforms to Freud's (1912) "unconscious-to-unconscious communication".

Bion's venture into epistemology, 1958–1967

As many outside the immediate circle of psychoanalysts were debating the validity of psychoanalysis (Hook, 1959; Popper, 1959; Grunbaum, 1984), and those inside were damning each other's perspectives, Bion – being no stranger to conflict – took up a question he never put down: What is psychoanalysis? He started a notebook of his reflections in 1958, and early in 1959 he wrote a long entry on R.B. Braithwaite's *Scientific Explanation* (Malin, 2021). He also adopted certain terminologies from the philosophy of science – "constant conjunction" (from David Hume), "scientific deductive system" (from Hempel), "elements" (from the idealist F.H. Bradley), and "selected fact" (from Henri Poincaré), among others. Clearly, Bion was attempting to establish psychoanalysis "as a natural science like any other", as Freud had put it (Freud, 1938, p. 158). By the mid-twentieth century, scientific criteria for validity had become much more rigorous.

Bion developed a complex paradigm for psychoanalytic "science", and even developed a grid of elements almost like Mendeleev's table of chemical elements. The exposition of this model was set out in two short, dense, and opaque texts – "Learning from Experience" and "Elements of Psychoanalysis" (Bion, 1962a, 1963). The model has been influential, and was responsible for a lot of subsequent speculation.

In a step intended to be helpful, he avoided terms which were already full of meaning (saturated, as he called them). In (relatively) simple terms, the maternal or caring (m)other is more than Freud's "object of an instinct" and is attributed another function beyond simple satisfaction or frustration. Like Winnicott's attempt to clothe the object in its own characteristic qualities, Bion found a specific function to the maternal carer. Mother is a potential container and has the task of taking on the infant's intolerable experiences herself. When a baby feels assaulted by experiences it cannot handle, it accumulates "beta-elements". This unsaturated term refers to experiences that cannot be graced by the term "meaningful" and which are felt like solid, even physical intrusions into the perceptual apparatus, eyes, ears, and so forth. Being quite unmanageable, they are then projected out as unwelcome or persecutory bits and pieces with the intention that the caring object take them in and make sense of them. If Klein assumed that the baby, from the beginning, is endowed only with a conception of a satisfying object or a frustrating one, Bion realised he had stumbled upon a possible third kind: an object that can make sense of, and know, experiences on behalf of the infant. This gives rise to three kinds of relation, referred to by Bion using the unsaturated symbols L, H, and K. The caring object has first to offer a receptivity, and then a making-sense function. He called making sense the "alpha-function"; it produces meaningful experiences out of the not yet meaningful, which he called alpha elements.

For Winnicott, as I understand it, "holding" is not yet meaning-making. Thus, the containing carer takes in the experience forced on them by the subject's intolerable panic, and that carer must rummage around among their own stock of experiences and memories to locate the closest meaning they can find to that which the infant has been defeated by. Alpha-function starts with a stock of pre-conceptions, then beta-elements (unprocessed perceptions) are introduced into the pre-conceptions and matched up more or less with one or another. When, in analysis, the matching is not so good, then part of the role of alpha-function is to reset the pre-conceptions to a greater or lesser degree for future encounters with experiences of the kind being dealt with. Once some matching/resetting had been achieved, the beta-element has been modified by being cloaked in some meaning or other, thus becoming an alpha-element. A simple example: the newborn baby cries due to some experience it has no meaning for, and this being a noxious experience, the baby can only conceive of the frustration as an attack that threatens survival, or something comparable. Mother is alarmed at her baby's screaming, but her stock of memories and pre-conceptions help her to realise that her baby is not being attacked or dying but needs to suckle and get some food. Mother has converted the intolerable sensations from the baby's tummy into a meaningful need – the beta-element has become an alpha-element with meaning. Moreover, the baby can achieve some new pre-conception for itself: the tummy feeling "means" a need for a nipple in the mouth.

All this is a rather meticulous and detailed pulling apart of the K kind of object-relation. It is important to note that this conforms to an idealism – following Kant's view that ideas are as important as the raw sense information in giving meanings. We are concerned with the ideas we accrue from our experiences. We do not see what is actually there (which would constitute realism). We see what our minds make of our perceptions; that is, we see appearances. This line of thinking progresses in a somewhat different direction from that of Freud (and perhaps of Winnicott).

Bion's two short books contributed nothing less than a Kleinian metapsychology running parallel to Freud's. However, Bion wanted more. His reading had taught him that for a science, a mathematical notation of neutral symbols set out in equations is necessary. His two epistemological books, *Learning from Experience* (Bion, 1962a) and *Elements of Psychoanalysis* (Bion, 1963), are laden with this mathematics-like notation. This he later dropped. In a further book, *Transformations*, published in 1965, he drew on a mathematical theory of transformations which says that things appear different from different perspectives. If you draw a circle on a piece of paper and then look at it from an angle, it appears as an ellipse. He applied this model to different perspectives in psychoanalysis.

According to the theory of transformations, something will look different from whatever perspective you take – both a circle and an ellipse are lines that enclose a space. This constant characteristic is called the "invariant". For example, Claude Monet painted a poppy field, but the painting is not the actual poppy field. There is one out there, and one that appeared to Monet's mind which he painted. There is an invariant – both are poppy fields. Whether actual or a representational, they are both poppy fields. It would seem Bion was understanding the way different psychoanalytic schools represent the same thing – their patients.

Representing, transforming, and communicating

We have gone a long way from the level of clinical paradigms, but Bion was never far removed from clinical thinking, no matter how abstract he got. His notion of transformation is relevant to the clinical setting; take an example he gives of a man greeting him when entering the consulting room:

> "Good morning, good morning, good morning. It must mean afternoon really. I don't expect anything can be expected today: this morning, I mean. This afternoon. It must be a joke of some kind. This girl left about her knickers. Well, what do you say to that? It's probably quite wrong, of course, but, well, I mean, what do *you* think?" He walked to the couch and lay down, bumping his shoulders down hard on the couch. "I'm slightly anxious…I think. The pain has come back in my knee. You'll probably say it was the girl. After all. This picture is probably not very good as I told him but I should not have said anything about it. Mrs. X…thought I ought to go to Durham to see about, but then" and so on.
>
> (Bion, 1965, pp. 143–144)

He then gave his own description of what the patient may have been feeling:

> He seemed as if he were pre-occupied with an object he had lost but expected to find close at hand. He corrected himself in a tone that might imply a mental aberration that had led him to think it "good morning". The speaker of the words "good morning", I gathered, was not really the patient, but someone whose manner he caricatured. Then came the comment that nothing could be expected. That was clear enough, but who was making the comment, or of whom nothing could be expected, was obscure. It might have been myself; I did not think it was he. Then he spoke of the joke. The way this term was used implied that the joke had no tincture of humour about it. To me it could mean a cruel joke, but such an interpretation depended on an assumption that the words retained the meaning that they would have in sane conversation and that the emotion expressed, by and with them, had the value that it would have in ordinary speech. When he spoke of "this" girl it was evident that I was supposed to know her; in fact I did not nor did I know whether she had left her knickers lying about or given notice on account of some episode connected with her knickers. "What do you say to that?" meant that in either case I would know as well as he did

> what her behaviour signified, though, as his next sentence showed, the significance (unmentioned) attached to her behaviour by both of us was probably mistaken, girls being what they are.
>
> (Bion, 1965, p. 20)

This second account attempts to give meaning to the patient's jumble of words. Bion is modest about his own interpretation, offering it in order to demonstrate how the analyst can produce something meaningful and communicable out of this meaningless utterance. The two accounts do not represent actual fact. The jumbled words of the patient can only be roughly transcribed. Bion thus gives an account from two perspectives: first his own (the analyst's), and second the patient's (as Bion imagines it). Two years later he wrote: "I do not regard any narrative purporting to be a report of fact, either of what the patient said or of what I said, as worth consideration as a 'factual account' of what happened" (Bion, 1967, p. 53) In fact, he conveyed that only two people could have anything valid to say about the material – the two who were there. From this point on, Bion's method of clinical reporting is extremely hesitant, as he attempted to return to the principle that the patient is the "fount of knowledge".

At this point, Bion is at another of his caesurae, and he disconcertingly changes direction. He drops his investigation of meaning-making (or alpha-function). Instead, he turns to an examination of the specific kind of communication that is involved, without making use of symbols.

Summary

The concept of holding describes the relation of a mother to her hardly conscious infant, who has no sense of self as yet. It involves the very bodily experience of being handled, and could be labelled love. Handling involves bringing a sense of a contact with another together with the experience of having a body, from which relation emerges a previously non-existent self. The phenomenon of being held by a mother creates the existence of the "Me", together with the alternative, the "Not-Me".

Despite the apparent similarity between Winnicott's "holding" and Bion's "containing", the latter is *not* about the coming into existence of the "Me", since for Bion, like Klein, the sense of a boundary between self and other exists from birth. Containing refers to the ability (or inability) to manage the experiences of the body or mind (initially the body). Containing is an important function (perhaps one not given to animals), involving managing these experiences, especially by creating a mental representation, typically in the form of words. Without these vitally important functions taking place between the infant and the other, the baby is "traumatised" (Winnicott) or suffers "nameless dread" (Bion). One might say that while Bion was concerned with meaning-making, Winnicott was attempting to understand self-making.

Despite the apparent similarity between holding and containing, there are more differences than might at first appear. Winnicott and Bion did both agree that physical, bodily care is experienced by the baby similarly to psychological care. In fact, the baby only distinguishes between bodily care and psychological love later. They also agreed on the importance of the quality of care for the baby. If this care is deficient, then for Winnicott the baby is at risk of losing the sense of a "continuity-of-being" and experience a passive collapse into a felt loss of identity and being. Bion, on the other hand, described a failure of containing as resulting in a worsening of the experience meant to be contained, a state he at one stage called "nameless dread": it results in a more specific disintegration initiated by the baby's ego itself, the aim being to split off the ego-function that generates the intolerable feeling.

Bion and Winnicott disagreed profoundly over one aspect of holding/containing. For Winnicott, the cause of any given problem is due to a failure on the part of the mother, who has full responsibility for providing benevolent physical and emotional holding. On the other hand, Bion regarded this relationship as more complex; it originates not with mother, but with the baby's experience of deprivation, need, or satisfaction, which are felt at first as bodily experiences. Noxious bodily experiences are then communicated, in the evocative/intuitive manner Bion emphasised, to the carer/mother, who has to be adequately receptive and fully experience that which the infant cannot tolerate. In the one case, the mother has to perform some sort of anticipatory function; in the other she must manage something intolerable.

Things can go wrong. In both conceptual models the mother/carer may fail, in which case, in Winnicott's conception, the baby sinks into a state of excessive "unthinkable agony"; in Bion's conception, the mother fails when she also experiences the baby's feelings as intolerable. In addition, for Bion, as development proceeds there is a reaction on the part of the baby to the carer, who is superior in their ability to tolerate and make sense of the intolerable – that is, what is intolerable for the baby demonstrates the baby's inadequacy and dependence and the carer's superior abilities. This developing awareness of the difference in adequacy can then lead to the baby conducting a destructive attack on the containing link (labelled, after Klein, as envy).

Bion grew very interested in the method of communication between baby and mother, which is clearly not language. It is much more akin to the calls of animals and birds, and has a direct evocative impact. The mother, and then the analyst, has to be especially prepared for receiving such communication. Winnicott similarly acknowledges a special receptivity in the mother that he named "primary maternal preoccupation", and he claimed that the analyst's capacity to "be" could offer the experience of "formlessness" that had not been afforded by the original object (that is, the mother). Similarly, Bion's model links maternal receptivity to analytic listening, which can be appreciated or attacked in the transference. Bion extended this to a recognition that the analyst's role, like the mother's, is to understand the state of mind and its intolerable experiences (he designated this "K"), while Winnicott emphasised the analyst's need to "be with" the patient's earliest traumatic experiences in order to work through early psychic deficiencies.

Table 3 Holding and containing

Winnicott	*Bion*
1. Mother's holding includes holding-the-baby-in-mind as well as the physical feeding, bathing and dressing	1. Bits of experience and of ego are projected into the analyst
2. Holding also integrates experience and develops the sense of "I am" (Me)	2. Experiences baby cannot handle accumulate as beta-elements
3. The mother adapts to her infant's needs	3. The maternal function is to make sense of, and know, experiences on behalf of the infant
4. Mother's empathy emanates from a deep identification with her infant	4. There is a non-symbolic form of communication typical of early infancy
5. The holding environment includes managing the baby's needs	5. Meaning-making is alpha-function
6. In depersonalisation, the individual experiences a mind-body split	6. The analyst sees and makes sense from a psychoanalytical perspective
8. Not-good-enough mothering traumatises the infant	
9. The analyst's attention and interpretative work constitutes the holding environment	
10. Being exists before doing and being-done-to	

Dialogue

Jan Abram: The comparisons between holding and containing as concepts from Winnicott and Bion respectively have indeed become very well known in the psychoanalytic literature and, to my mind, are often misconstrued. As I said in Chapter 5, Winnicott's concept of holding is often misunderstood and seen as less complex than Bion's concept of container-contained. I think you make the same mistake in your Chapter 6 when you suggest that "holding is not yet meaning-making". I hope that in this dialogue we can begin to clarify each concept in order to show how they sometimes overlap and make clear the distinctions where they are different. Hopefully our chapters will stimulate questions from both of us as well as our readers. Let me start with some thoughts I have from the beginning of your chapter.

I was very struck that, from your point of view, Bion was "released" after 1960 to formulate a Kleinian metapsychology. You seem to infer that after the death of Melanie Klein, Bion felt freer to formulate a new Kleinian model. This resonated with a view I came to during my research on Winnicott's work as I was preparing *The Language of Winnicott* in the early 1990s. At first I found that Winnicott's writings seemed to flourish in the early 1960s. Although he was clearly building on his previous theories, his language and approach manifested a sense of freedom in his thought, and his work during his late years is inspiring as well as consolidating. I became very curious about why this occurred specifically after 1960. When I realised that Melanie Klein had died that year, it seemed clear that this may well have made a difference to Winnicott's sense of freedom, which manifests as a freedom of thought. This is hypothetical of course. But it makes me wonder about both Winnicott and Bion's transference to Melanie Klein, which, in part, was perpetuated by the conviction she had about her evolving theories.

I'm reminded of a paper Winnicott presented to the British Society on 7 January 1948 in which he proposes that a child is vulnerable to a parent's depression to the extent that their own personal sense of guilt is not recognised intrapsychically. He gives some clinical examples before he applies this theory to the institutional factor and how these themes are played out in any given group. He picks up on Edward Glover's papers of 1945 and 1949 in which he (Glover) expresses that Klein and her pupils describe certain fantasies of their patients' which really belong to themselves (the analysts). Winnicott poses an essential question that concerns new ideas in psychoanalysis and suggests that a clear distinction needs to be retained between the value of ideas and the feelings that are aroused by them because of the way they are presented. Here, it seems apparent that Winnicott was expressing his opinion that Klein's concept of the "depressive position" was valuable but, at the same time, the way in which it was introduced expressed a militancy which could potentially spoil the value of the concept.

This is an example of Winnicott's response to the Controversial Discussions again, and I think it's inevitable that we return to the conflicts and the fallout from those conflicts during this period in the history of the British Psychoanalytical Society. I think it is clear that Winnicott valued many of Klein's contributions but was dismayed by the way her work was promoted by her followers. This "militant" approach to psychoanalytic ideas and concepts goes against the grain of psychoanalysis – something that we are trying to avoid throughout this book, especially in the dialogues. I think we may agree so far on the above and on the beginning of your Chapter 6.

Let me comment on your section "Briefly from the 1950s". It seems to me that in this short paragraph the real differences between the concepts – holding and containing – come to light.

Firstly, let me address the use of language in Kleinian theory. I've always found it rather alienating and mechanical, although, as you know, I've also found your dictionary on Kleinian thought very helpful for appreciating the meaning behind the sometimes off-putting language (Hinshelwood, 1989).

The term "projective identification" is unnecessarily clunky in my view. It complicates rather than clarifies what occurs between parent and infant. You suggest that Bion wished to elaborate on this concept of Klein's by making what she suggested was pathological (that is, projective identification) into something that Bion suggested was also a "kind of communication" – and therefore something normal. This became – I think you suggest – Bion's theory of communication. I will return to this point on Winnicott's theory of communication, but first let me comment on the language Bion uses and what I feel it conveys.

I appreciate that you are citing these paragraphs as a way of examining what Bion proposed about the operation of container-contained. Firstly, we hear that the patient needs to "rid himself of the fear of death" by "splitting off his fears and putting them into his analyst". I am interested in trying to see the theories that underlie this sentence. There seems to me to be an underlying assumption that the patient's fear of death exists because the infant is born with an innate death instinct which causes the fear of death right from the start. Winnicott did not agree with Klein's version of the death instinct. He also disagreed with Freud's concept of the death instinct. I think both concepts, Freud's and Klein's, are different, although they use the same term.

Winnicott suggested that the newborn infant is not capable of knowing or feeling a fear of death. At the very start, the infant is not able to distinguish between life and death. At the earliest stage the infant is inevitably caught up with surviving. This is very different from a concept of fear of anything, I think. I'm sure Winnicott's concept is much more closely related to Freud's notion of the instinct of survival (that is, the self preservative instinct).

The other basic assumption seems to me to be that the analyst has a psyche that will modify the patient's fear (of death) as long as the projections have a chance to "repose" in the analyst's psyche. This assumption seems to me to ascribe omnipotence to the analyst.

I find the language used about the patient infers a kind of intentionality on the patient's part, even though I assume (although I have no way of knowing) that Bion did not really wish to convey that.

Then we have the reference to what the mother "should" have done for her infant. And here we have Bion's elaboration of Klein's view, in which he brings in the environment and what the environment/mother needs to do for the infant. There is an assumption that the baby will begin fearing death as soon as they are born. The mother needs to "experience the feeling of dread", and it is her ability to experience this that makes her the container – but only if she can truly "experience this feeling of dread".

The main points of disagreement between Winnicott and Bion are the assumption that all newborn infants experience a fear of death and that the analyst's psyche has the power to change that "split-off" fear so that the patient will be able to re-introject or take in the mother's capacity to tolerate the fear of dying.

I'll briefly mention how Winnicott theorises what happens to the infant in his theory of holding. Firstly, from the beginning of his work, Winnicott was formulating a theory of communication that reached its zenith in 1963 in "Communicating and not communicating leading to a study of certain opposites". The mother who is able to hold her infant goes into a state of primary maternal preoccupation based on her deep identification with the baby's sense of helplessness and need to survive. It is through handling the infant, speaking to the infant verbally and non-verbally, and being totally engaged with tasks that are both physiological and psychological that she mediates all the infant's feelings. If, and only if, she is able to carry out these tasks emotionally and physically – but mostly emotionally – will the baby then be able to feel that its needs are being adapted to; in turn, the mother survives due to her reliability and lack of retaliation for whatever the baby causes her in the way of suffering. In his late work, Winnicott outlined the five stages of the mother-infant interaction in his paper "The use of an object" (Winnicott, 1969a).

In Winnicott's theory, the analyst is able to offer something the original mother was not: the analyst is able to psychically survive, and it is this different response to the patient that makes all the difference therapeutically. Winnicott's stress on playing and following the patient's communications makes the analytic encounter much more about co-creativity between patient and analyst than about the analyst doing something to or for the patient. The analyst, like the mother who is able to mediate the infant's feelings, follows the patient's communications in a radically different way from the mother who could not carry out this task for whatever reason. This is the therapeutic action of psychoanalysis.

Robert D. Hinshelwood: I think you get to the nub of it with your last sentence – the nature of the therapeutic action of psychoanalysis. What we think of therapeutic "action" has changed since Freud interpreted dreams, hasn't it? A key paper was Strachey's in 1934, when Winnicott finished his analysis with Strachey and looked for a Kleinian analyst – rightly or wrongly.

Bion explicitly set out the steps in therapeutic action. It would be helpful, perhaps, if Winnicott's model of development could be put in that same step-by-step form. Bion's steps were: (i) a subject has an intolerable and incomprehensible experience; (ii) this is communicated (non-symbolically) to another; (iii) the other receives the direct communication of the actual experience as a replica in themselves (not as a representation); (iv) the other recognises it as some sort of experience which does have a comprehensible meaning and (v) communicates that back to the subject in a symbolic verbal form; then, in addition, (vi) the subject acquires in the process a function by which they can, in the future, recognise that comprehension which the other has given to the experience.

It is important that Bion saw this first and foremost as a transaction of the adult with his/her analyst. He did indeed apply this as a theory of development in the infant. However, neither Bion nor anyone else can claim to know exactly, what the experiences or understandings of an infant are. And Bion would be the last person to think that a fear of death as we comprehend it as a adults is comparable to a baby's experience.

For a start, most adults do have a comprehension of some kind of experience that they expect to be the experience of death. That comprehension varies among us, and it is seriously complicated by religious beliefs, some of which may be acceptable because they ameliorate the dread. Nevertheless, there is some deep-down dread in all of us that goes back a long way. It is not graced with the verbal symbol "death", but it does explain why horror films are a great draw and frequently make for box-office successes, and why crime thrillers usually have a corpse as their centrepiece. The dread and the need to give it some comprehensibility probably remain a lifelong pre-occupation.

I am sure you are right that the infant's incomprehensible experience does not compare much with an adult's attempts to comprehend it. Maybe Winnicott's term "surviving" is most appropriate. I think perhaps it does not really matter what we call it, as whatever term we use seems inevitably to deny the quality of incomprehension. For an infant encountering an experience for the first time, it must inevitably be impossible to comprehend it. It is only later, when the baby and its experiences are handled by an understanding parent, that some elements of comprehension evolve.

Of course, in the first instance, the mother-baby interaction regarding the incomprehensible has to be non-verbal and, we could assume, non-symbolic. It has to be communicated in action. If a baby feels hungry for the first time, it must alert its mother to do something about it. And as you say, mother is the one who must understand and enact something that "does the trick". She does do something, she feeds. And her feeding is at the same time a communication. It is an action that says (without words), "When you have that feeling, you want me to feed you".

Bion was interested in this earliest of developmental processes, but specifically as it emerges in adult life. It is a process that goes on all of our lives. Perhaps for every funeral we go to we gain a slightly greater comprehension of dying. But this does not dislodge the earliest feeling of dread; it merely makes it more comprehensible in some way. And Aristotle might agree that this is the function of tragedy in theatre. This is different from Freud, and I suspect from Winnicott. For Freud, the earliest qualities are pleasure and unpleasure (or pain), but Bion wanted to establish that, for the human at least, these early and perhaps innate experiences, pleasure and unpleasure, quickly become supplemented by the qualities of comprehension and incomprehension. In his irritating (and not completely successful way), Bion liked to reduce these ideas to a notation. Where, as he said, pleasure and unpleasure can be referred to as "L" and "H", respectively, there is also "K". In this, Bion was a Kleinian, since Klein's earliest papers on observing children concerned their ability to grasp the facts of life and the obstructions to their grasping them – in effect, K is Freud's epistemophilic component of the libido.

What has greatly expanded this meaning-making process is the human invention of symbols, especially verbal ones. From early on, and perhaps since he studied Kant at Oxford in 1920, Bion was interested in the way we give sense and meaning to the objects behind the experiences we receive from our perceptual senses, the "thing-in-itself". This huge human expansion of meaning-making is our cultural heritage, the compound total of all those appearances. However, it is also the case that we never leave behind that primary experience of pleasure-unpleasure. That dimension, the pleasure principle of Freud, is for Bion (as for Freud) binary. Bion says that we must comprehend satisfaction and frustration as well as feel them; and more, he says that the human mind can make frustration a degree more tolerable through an act of comprehension or meaning-making.

The issue we end up arguing about is what Bion and Winnicott regarded the pole the Freud called "unpleasure". We cannot know the exact experience, only its derivatives, which arrive much later (conceived of as horror films, for instance). There is no reason to throw out the terms "fear of survival" or "death instinct". They are both terms, symbols, words, and therefore they have already disposed of the essential quality for the infant – the incomprehensibility of the experience – by symbolising it in a word.

Neither Bion nor Winnicott deny the existence of the negative pole of the pleasure principle; they do acknowledge that negative state, whether it is called a feeling of death or of non-survival. Both terms are symbols and miss the essential quality. Does "dread" come nearer to it? Perhaps only aesthetic creativity can begin to evoke the incomprehensible quality.

I have not dealt with all your points, but I hope that by distinguishing pleasure-unpleasure from comprehension-incomprehension we can enrich the dimensions in which we compare Bion with Winnicott. It is comprehension which is the therapeutic action.

J.A.: You seem to be saying that you think the "therapeutic action" of psychoanalysis changed since Freud's interpretation of dreams and that this change was instigated by James Strachey's classic paper "On the therapeutic action of psychoanalysis" (Strachey, 1934). Perhaps we would both agree today that Strachey's systematic outline of psychoanalytic technique (which includes the moment of urgency and the mutative interpretation) is at the very heart of technique for the majority of British trained psychoanalysts. I might even venture to suggest that it could be the one paper that, no matter what theoretical orientation their analytic work is based on, brings the majority of analysts together. However, the way in which technique has evolved, and is still evolving since Strachey's paper, differs according to the various orientations, and I think you show this when you finish by saying that "it is comprehension which is the therapeutic action". You imply here that once the patient "understands" their unconscious, they are cured. I realise I'm stating this rather boldly and possibly simplistically, but perhaps you could elaborate on this point? I know that in Part V we will be looking much more closely at technique and the differences between Winnicott and Bion, but your response would be helpful as it will lead into Part V.

I'd like to briefly elaborate on my statement about the commonality of technique in the British Psychoanalytical Society. Of course, I have to warn the reader that this is my particular view. For the past few years I have convened a course for the MSc on Psychoanalytic Studies at University College London – Contemporary Clinical Theory. For each seminar, a senior analyst of the British Society presents on the way they work according to their theoretical orientation. The analyst presents the theories according to their own model, whether Kleinian, Contemporary Freudian, or Independent. Each model is quite distinct, and yet when it comes to technique, the common denominator is the transference and countertransference. Briefly, each school has their own theoretical emphasis, and each analyst selects certain papers that have meaning for them. But when listening to the discussion of clinical work, the emphasis on process and the evolving transference is what brings each school together. Nevertheless, each school has a kind of hallmark. The Kleinian tends to intervene more, and each intervention is an interpretation of the transference. The Contemporary Freudian will listen more and tends to pace their interventions in order to check whether they feel the patient is "ready" for the interpretation. The Independent tends to listen for the infantile layers of the narrative and how they manifest in the transference. I won't elaborate further in this dialogue, as I will do so in Chapter 9 of Part V. My point here, just to clarify, is that each different emphasis, while working in the transference, is founded on a basic assumption. That is what we are trying to examine by asking the question: Does this matter or not in the final analysis? I will return to this.

Let me now return to Winnicott and Bion. I was very struck that you said that Bion "would be the last person to think that a fear of death as we comprehend it as adults is comparable to a baby's experience". Later you say that "maybe Winnicott's term 'surviving' is better", and you go on to say that it doesn't really matter what we call it. This surprised me, because when I have had conversations with other Kleinians, most of them have been convinced that the infant is born into the world with the problem of anxiety caused by the innate death instinct. This is a very different perspective from that of Winnicott, who insists that the infant is born into the world with "inherited tendencies" that require mediating by the mother, who has the ability to recognise the precariousness of the early moments/ hours/days/weeks. The fact of dependence makes for a different theoretical approach to the fact of the death instinct. I know we have discussed this in our first book, but it does need to be reiterated in relation to Bion, who as you confirm was certainly a Kleinian.

So I think it does matter very much, Bob, how we conceptualise early development and how it manifests itself in the analysing situation, which mobilises a variety of infantile layers, hidden and repressed in each adult analysand.

Meanwhile, I appreciate the notion of meaning-making and the need to experience frustration and satisfaction as well as to understand them. However, I think Winnicott was much more interested in formlessness and being. Without the experience of being at the start of life, the baby is not going to be able to comprehend other than through a split in the intellect.

R.D.H.: Let's clarify the Strachey paper: I think it was a distinct landmark in 1934. However, the idea of interpreting parental imagoes is a bit different from interpreting instinctual cathexes as the Viennese were beginning to do. The Viennese in the 1930s were increasingly interested in the ego's ability to confront the power of the instincts, their repression with counter-cathexes, their sublimation, and so on. But this of course was developed especially strongly and in a detailed fashion when they got to the US after 1938 as the school of ego-psychology. The British analysts at the time Bion was training, from 1938 to 1950 (interrupted by the Second World War), were less interested in the ego as the controller of the instincts and more as it is composed of relations with objects and identifications with them. They were interested in the people we relate to in the mind, important figures who we might have imaginary conversations with and who do not exist for the moment in our external word. It was a focus developing in parallel to (and partly growing out of) Freud's description of the super-ego as an internal entity in relation to the ego. So Strachey represented that specific British orientation.

About the therapeutic action, I think it is important to develop an understanding of therapeutic action in Bion's thinking. He was interested in "knowing" as a mental function – and even used a cipher, K, for it – as well as the resistance to knowing – minus-K. In fact, he set K alongside loving and hating as the three primary modalities of relating between people. This is a very complex issue to get into, and it has a deep philosophical tinge. Remember, Bion studied philosophy at Oxford after the First World War, some ten years before he became a doctor and then a psychoanalyst, as mentioned previously. He was influenced by the Kantian scholar H.J. Paton. Crucial here is the Kantian idea that we never know exactly what we perceive, only our interpretations. We do not see wavelengths of light, we see green or red. In effect we see appearances – the way things appear to us when we have processed them, such as the three-dimensional template we use of space. At one point Bion likened it to the optical illusion wherein one can see two faces or alternatively the shape of a vase.

I am not sure how fundamental this is to Winnicott (in Chapter 1 you quote his 1960 paper). For Bion, we know very little of our reality except from the way we experience it. This is known as an idealist philosophy; we see things in terms of the ideas we have (this was developed as phenomenology). It differs from a positivist philosophy wherein there is a much greater confidence that we know things as they are (not as we construct them). Freud separated these two kinds of perceptions into the pleasure principle and the reality principle as a developmental sequence. Freud never put it like that, and it is a rather slick correlation perhaps. As infants, we experience what we perceive in terms of what we want and what we are denied – only subsequently can we begin to know things more as they really are.

It seems to me that Winnicott is much more of a positivist than Bion. Winnicott seems to think that from the beginning the infant can know the reality of a mother who is or is not good enough. For Bion (following Klein), as infants we know "mother" in terms of how we process the experience of her. For the very young infant, the world is populated by starkly different and polarised others. Mother is a loved and loving object when she satisfies, and a hated and hateful object when she does not. Only later can the infant begin to recognise the reality of a mixed kind of figure more akin to a mother who satisfies and frustrates at different moments. I wonder if this underlying diversity of philosophical premises helps to locate some of the difference.

Yes, of course, I take your point that we are each telling our own stories here. But I very much doubt if there are many who assert a death instinct in the manner of Freud's idea of entropy. Or perhaps I should say, Kleinians do not think of an innate death instinct any more than an innate libido; or perhaps to put it the other way, there is as much innate libido as innate death instinct. The point is that both death instinct and libido are provoked/stimulated by the external object that delivers satisfaction or frustration. They are seen as deeply polarised, as I suggest, at the most infantile level (or in Klein's terms, at the deepest levels of the unconscious in the here and now). I think your experience of listening to analysts of different persuasions is interesting. A systematic set of alternative assumptions would be very helpful to have. In particular, who assumes transference is a strict continuity with the infant from the past rather than an active infantile level now? Who assumes an accurate assessment of the infant's external object and who an infantile external object constructed from innate and given experiences of satisfaction/frustration? There may be a research project there!

I think I need to hear more about the variation in the innate or inherited tendencies of infants. Of course it is true that we cannot know for certain, can we? We can only make inferences. But nevertheless I am not sure of the difference in substance between the two assumptions. You say there is a very great difference between an infant "born into the world with the problem of anxiety caused by the innate death instinct" and an infant "born into the world with 'inherited tendencies' that require mediating by the mother, who has the ability to recognise the precariousness". I wonder if you can elaborate on the difference, although I agree the words used are very different. For instance, a fear for survival and precariousness appear to be different words, but point in very much the same direction.

I do agree that how we see the early infant is important because of the way such models inform the present. I want to move away from talking about Kleinians. Bion, though he was a Kleinian, was never a child therapist/paediatrician, and his formative experiences were with adults in groups. The early infantile situation was not of great interest to him, as he was interested in what was "primitive" in the present. Bion, to my knowledge, never used the term "death instinct", so we might want to leave that aside for our present dialogues. He developed his clinical work in the 1950s, when the Kleinians became interested in investigating envy as a destructive and self-destructive set of impulses that wreck the coherence of the self (ego) and arouse powerful guilt and concern for the envied other. It is loosely connected with the death instinct as a destructive force provoked by (largely) external circumstances that are there in reality or which have been internalised. Bion developed his idea of envy in a paper read to the society in 1957, the year Klein's little book, *Envy and Gratitude,* was published.

His paper "Attacks on linking", published in 1959, was very clear about the attacking destructiveness. Attacks were made on the *link* with an object that was potentially of use. Somewhat later than Bion, Hanna Segal defined envy in this way: "Envy is described by Melanie Klein…as a spoiling hostility at the realization that the source of life and goodness lies outside" (Segal, 1983, p. 270). So, for Segal, envy and narcissism are intimately connected – "Two sides of the same coin", she said.

Bion's version is more specific. In line with the points made earlier in this part of the book, Bion described the innate need for meaning-making and how the infant with a primary love-hate polarity needs an external object to moderate such meanings and make them more applicable to reality. This is the specific role of the external object. It has to help to make the infant's experiences meaningful in a way that allows the meanings to become useable in reality. This, for Bion, is a primary K link, and it is an intimate one between the self and other. For this dependence, the other reaps the hatred of narcissism. Bion's understanding of destructiveness is the product of his work with colleagues, but his version is very specific and became more detailed in subsequent published work.

Finally, I wonder if you could specify the therapeutic action of the holding process in the step-by-step way that Bion described containing. Or will it not admit such a descriptive process?

J.A.: Thank you, Bob – yes, it's helpful to bear in mind the history of the evolving psychoanalytic theories post WW2, especially in relation to the USA and London. As I previously said, I do think that despite the difference in the theoretical underpinnings in London, most British analysts work in the transference along object-relation lines. However, the stress placed on interpreting aggression is very much a Kleinian emphasis. That is not to say that Independents and Contemporary Freudians are not aware of aggression, hate, and envy especially. But it does seem to be a matter of emphasis for them. If the (Kleinian) analyst believes that envy in the patient is the most toxic emotion, I suppose they would wish to interpret this affect for the patient's own good. But interpreting unconscious envy may alienate many patients who are not ready to look at their most negative affects, and interpretations can often sound very accusing, to patients as well as to analysts listening to clinical material, with a lot of interpretations being aimed at the patient's envy. What you highlight and cite from Hannah Segal, for example, illustrates a particular belief that all analysands will inevitably be envious of their analyst because, according to this theory, de facto, analysts are the source of life and goodness. From what you say, Bion had a more heuristic view of psychoanalysis, and this is where Winnicott and Bion have much in common – especially when you say Bion's primary K link places the responsibility for the infant's development on the mother. Although I think Winnicott's emphasis was much more on how the infant and mother played together. Nevertheless, it's true to say that Winnicott does place the mother at the centre of the infant's development because she has a maturity the infant does not.

You're right to point out the differences between Winnicott's background in medicine and paediatrics and Bion's background in philosophy (noting especially the Kantian notion of perception). Winnicott was rather derogatory about philosophy. He once wrote towards the end of his life:

> We could use a Frenchified word *existing* and talk about existence, and we can make this into a philosophy and call it existentialism, but somehow or other we like to start with the word *being* and then with the statement *I am*.
>
> (Winnicott, 1966, p. 11 – 12, in Abram, 2007 p. 68)

Funnily enough though, it is the French analysts who have embraced Winnicott's work since the 1960s, because, despite Winnicott's dislike of philosophy, his writings have a philosophical depth – especially in his late work, as seen in *Playing and Reality* (1971a). This takes me on to my response to your not being sure how fundamental the notion of perception was to Winnicott. Actually it became fundamental in his late work, as seen in "The use of an object" (Winnicott, 1969a), in which he wishes to delineate how the infant moves from apperception to perception. Chapter 7 is where I will go into more detail about this. I'm struck that you mention Freud's, 1911 paper on the "Formulation of the two principles of mental functioning" as a separation of two kinds of perception – pleasure and reality principles – because I've long thought that Winnicott's "The use of an object" is a development of and even an advance on that paper. So this is all to say that, yes, Winnicott was very interested in perception and how it developed. I want to add, therefore, that I don't think your take on Freud's 1911 paper is "slick".

But I'm afraid I do wish to correct you on another point you make about Winnicott when you say that the baby "knows" whether the mother is good enough or not. On the contrary, Winnicott's point about the very beginning is that due to the infant's unawareness (that is, apperception – his term for the state of mind before the development of the ability to perceive, when there is a merger between subject and object), as long as the mother *is* good enough, the baby can start to emerge out of the merger and move from object-relating to object usage, which defines the journey from unawareness to awareness – Me and Not-Me. A baby who is traumatised for whatever reason does not know the environment is bad at the time of being traumatised. The only defence the baby has at the earliest stage of development is to withdraw (Winnicott, 1952; Abram and Hinshelwood, 2018). So, coming from very different backgrounds, it would seem that Bion's perspective is in line with Winnicott's regarding what the baby has to come to terms with.

I don't think you're right to assume that many analysts do not follow Freud's death instinct. There are many who do amongst the Contemporary Freudians and French psychoanalysis (see especially Perelberg, 2015). But let me just respond to your questions related to assumptions about the transference. I can't think that any psychoanalyst would say that the past comes into the transference "strictly" from the "actual" real situation. Psychoanalysis is all about how we interpret our past, isn't it? I think we said this in a previous dialogue (perhaps in the IPA webinar). It's always what the individual "makes" of the past. You and Bion would say this is Kantian?

You end your response by asking me if I could specify the therapeutic action of the holding process in the step-by-step way that Bion described containing. I do this in Chapter 7, which takes us naturally into Part IV of our book. Are we ready now to go on to that part?

R.D.H.: Thanks for the final bit of dialogue. I am happy to go on with Part IV. But I am not sure that we have gotten to the necessary depth of understanding of what interpretation is or does. And maybe it will become central in Part IV, as you say. The necessary interpretation is not so much about interpreting the envy as such, but rather about the care and regret and concern for the object that is envied (as well as needed and loved as the source of life). I believe Winnicott absolutely agreed with this, didn't he? After all, Winnicott and Klein were good colleagues in the mid-1930s, when Klein was developing all this.

But we are actually more interested in Bion now, and how he took off from Klein's paranoid-schizoid position – Bion was deeply involved in understanding the weakening and loss of the sense of self. And it is very regrettable that he and Winnicott were not able to acknowledge each other's work in this direction. So Bion's approach to envy would entail that the way of dealing with it is to dismantle the ego that can feel envy, ending up with a dismantled ego.

Perhaps all this will come out in Part IV. I will now go on to read your Chapter 7.

PART **IV**

CONSOLIDATION AND NEW BEGINNINGS

Chapters 7 and 8 present the contrasting ways Winnicott and Bion developed, with reference to the apparent interconnections between their new formulations. Certain concepts seemed to overlap, but without mutual acknowledgement and dialogue.

DOI: 10.4324/9781003382409-11

CHAPTER SEVEN

From primary maternal preoccupation to the use of an object

Jan Abram

This chapter outlines the late concepts of Winnicott and examines the minute details of the earliest psychic development that stem from his early work on the maternal. During this late period, it is the nature of the mother's contribution that makes all the difference to the nascent psyche.

Ordinary devotion

Through his work as a paediatrician Winnicott was in a position to consult hundreds of mothers and infants over several decades. This meant that from early on in his work he became aware of the ordinary mother's devotion towards their infants. The term "ordinary devotion" originated in 1949, when Winnicott was discussing with a BBC producer what to call the series of nine lectures he was going to give on the radio (Abram, 2007, p. 259). This is an example of how Winnicott invented new terms that capture succinctly the psychology of the mother with her new born infant. He recognised that "ordinarily" the woman enters a phase just before she is going to give birth wherein she occupies a state of mind in which she becomes completely preoccupied with the infant because of her intense identification with the infant's state of helplessness. By 1956, the concept

DOI: 10.4324/9781003382409-12

of "primary maternal preoccupation" had evolved out of his observations of ordinary devotion.

Through her unconscious memories, the mother is able to enter into this state of mind, and when the time is appropriate, she recovers from the state as it becomes clear that the infant can start to separate. Most mothers do not recognise this state of mind as they are caught up in the momentum necessary to maintain it. Winnicott said that the mother's response comes about because "she was a baby once" and therefore has a deep-seated experience of being cared for (or not). The unconscious memories instate a kind of deep identification that is transmitted from mother to infant and which in turn facilitates the mother's ability to hold and handle the baby and to be in tune with the infant's needs. Primary maternal preoccupation is a necessary state of mind in order for the mother to be able to adapt to the infant's needs.

Winnicott also wished to emphasise that he was identifying a developmental process between the infant and their mother that is distinct from anything previously proposed. He went so far as to suggest that if it were not for the baby's existence, the mother's state of mind would be likened to a psychiatric condition. While he confirmed it is an "organised state", it can simultaneously be compared with a dissociated state or a fugue or "even with a disturbance at a deeper level such as a schizoid episode" (Winnicott, 1958).

Meeting the infant's needs is not possible without the mother's unconditional love. She is merged with her infant through her deep identification. In order to surrender to this state of mind, the mother of the newborn needs all the holding she can get from her emotional and physical environment (that is, her family members, especially the baby's father).

The outcome for the infant is that a sense of continuity-of-being is set up at a deep level of psychological functioning. I think the reader will see clearly that primary maternal preoccupation is absolutely necessary in order for the infant to feel loved through being rocked, held, and named in the loving arms of a mother who is completely taken over by this essential task. At this stage the mother and infant are psychologically merged. During this phase there are no object relations yet, only ego support from mother to infant and ego-relatedness from infant to mother.

This 1958 paper was a highly original contribution to perinatal care management. Several years later, in 1968, arising out of this formulation, Winnicott, for the first time, was able to define the stages of exchange that resolve the problem of defining the details of what he came to describe as the process of "object relating to object usage".

The use of an object

Alongside his work as a paediatrician, Winnicott saw children, adolescents, and adults in his private psychoanalytic practice. This complementary work informed his far-reaching advances in psychoanalysis practice and theory, and his work is increasingly recognised as having created a new and different clinical paradigm from that of both Freud and Klein. This means that his focus, especially in his late work, was on introducing several notions that many authors have suggested advance the theory and practice of psychoanalysis (see Abram, 2013; Ogden, 2022).

Winnicott proposed that the core problem for the human being is not primarily psychosexuality, as Freud held; nor is it the death instinct or aggression, as was suggested by Klein and Bion; rather it is the "fact of dependency". This observation shifted the focus in psychoanalysis to the early psychic primary relationship. Subjectivity, in this paradigm, is inscribed with the mother's primary maternal preoccupation (or not).

A close examination of Winnicott's theoretical advances reveal that their foundations reside firmly with Freud such that human nature can only be examined and experienced through the lens of Freud's clinical methodology and its therapeutic aims. By recognising different stages of dependency related to the early maternal holding environment, Winnicott's clinical investigations led to an extension of Freud's concept of *hilflosigkeit* (helplessness). But primary aggression in the newborn was, for Winnicott, benign primary creativity.

I have elsewhere suggested that *survival-of-the-object* is at the heart of Winnicott's clinical-theoretical paradigm, whereby he determined that the mother's role shapes the nascent psyche rather than instincts.

"The instincts can be as much external as can a clap of thunder or a hit"

What interests Winnicott above all is how the baby is able to make the intrapsychic move from object-relating to the use of an object. This was his lifelong quest, and in 1970, several months before he died, he wrote that he had identified the essential ingredient in early psychic development and had therefore solved the problem of the "crude primitive excited idea" when he wrote "The use of an object". I previously suggested that his solution lay in identifying the role of the mother, who facilitates the infant's psychic movement from object-relating to object survival; from apperception to perception; from pre-ruth to ruth.

The Mother's role in relating to her infant involves a five-stage sequence in early object-relating.

A dissection of the sequence

1. *Subject relates to object*

This depicts the mother's profound attention (primary maternal preoccupation) and the baby who is merged with her during the phase of absolute dependence.

2. *Object is in process of being found instead of placed by the subject in the world*

The baby's needs are being met and this "adaptation to needs" leads to a glimmer of awareness of the object.

3. *Subject destroys object*

The baby's repeated and uninhibited ruthless demand for the mother's adaptation to their needs amounts to a continual destruction of the object. This is a necessary process of discovering the externality of the mother.

4. *Object survives destruction*

The mother's sustained capacity to tolerate the baby's endless demands because of her state of primary maternal preoccupation offers the infant a sense of continuity-of-being. Survival involves primary identification, mirroring, ego protection, and, essentially, *non*-retaliation. The myriad aspects of the mother's psychic survival facilitate the infant's movement from apperception to perception in the potential space between relating to subjective objects and perceiving objects objectively perceived.

5. *Subject can use object*

The previous merger of the environment mother and object mother in the phase of absolute dependence gave the impression to the infant that there were two different mothers. Due to the consistent *survival-of-the-object*, this perspective has gradually changed, and by now the baby is able to see that both mothers are actually one.

The "new feature" was introduced for the first time in 1968, to a New York audience (see Abram, 2013, ch. 14). After the subject relates to the object comes the subject's destruction of the object (as it becomes external); and then may come "object survives destruction by the subject". A new feature thus arrives in the theory of object relating.

> The subject says to the object: I destroyed you, and the object is there to receive the communication. From now on the subject says: Hello Object. I destroyed you. I love you. You have value for me because of your survival of my destruction of you. While I am loving you I am all the time destroying you in unconscious fantasy. Here fantasy begins for the individual. The subject can now use the object that has survived.
>
> (Winnicott, 1969a)

Let me emphasise here that the subject can now use the object because of the maternal psychic *survival-of-the-object* (Abram, 2022).

CHAPTER EIGHT

Rethinking and making an impact

R.D. Hinshelwood

Bion's progress was erratic (see Hinshelwood, 2022). Having decided there was a crisis over how to transcend the different perspectives represented by the analyst and the analysand, he began to focus on the method of listening. Most of his theoretical, or epistemological, work of the early 1960s seemed to be redundant and gradually faded from his interest.

Dealing with pre-conceptions

Bion remained committed to the intuitive introspective method and his Kantian idealism. The issue for him was how to find a position in which his own need to make sense using his pre-conceptions did not interfere too much with the patient's way of making sense with their own pre-conceptions. This also resonated with the need for analysts to put down their pre-conceived theories when debating with each other.

At first, he announced his intention to abandon memory and desire and to treat each new session as if it were with a completely new patient altogether (Bion, 1965). When he gave a brief account of this during his seminars in Los Angeles in 1967, it was roundly criticised by several commentators as naïve (Aguayo and Malin 2013). Analysts build up a

 DOI: 10.4324/9781003382409-13

picture of their patients' internal world and unconscious phantasies over time – and they (the analyst) need to remember over time. Moreover, the idea that one can consciously control the determinants of one's conscious thinking by stopping one's own memories and desires is not very psychoanalytic, since we assume that everything is highly determined by unconscious factors.

Nevertheless, Bion had not meant it naïvely, since he was intent on understanding how to manage one's own receptivity, or reverie as he now called it, and to keep it as clear as possible from one's own interfering preconceptions. This was a genuine issue of central importance and he gradually came to a more sophisticated appreciation of what he was trying to get at.

In *Transformations* (Bion, 1965) he took the idea of the "invariant" as important. The invariant underlies all perspectives and is what is transformed by everyone's own point of view. With his interest in notation, he gave this invariant the symbol "O", and there has been an enormous amount of subsequent literature on the subject. It equates with the Kantian thing-in-itself, which is not known directly but which lies behind the appearances we each fashion from our perceptions. The challenge, therefore, is to know what lies behind our worked-up perception. At this point, Bion turned to his interest in intuition and the capacity for receiving a direct kind of impact. Bion spent the rest of his career working out if direct intuition could be a means of communicating the invariant. Psychoanalysis takes as its focus the patient's experience, which is thus the invariant for us all.

Non-sensuous perceptions

Bion attempted to characterise this direct intuitive impact in his book *Attention and Interpretation* (1970):

> The physician can see and touch and smell. The realizations with which a psycho-analyst deals cannot be seen or touched; anxiety has no shape or colour, smell or sound. For convenience, I propose to use the term "intuit" as a parallel in the psychoanalyst's domain to the physician's use of "see", "touch", "smell", and "hear".
>
> (Bion, 1970, p. 7)

So, anxiety can be indicated in pallor, physical tension, and so forth, but what we know of the other person is that they are anxious. When someone else is anxious, we simply "know" their anxiety and feel it in ourselves, although we also know that what we feel is not our own anxiety but theirs. We intuit by harbouring the feeling within us.

Bion was separating two modes of communication – communication by representation in symbols, typically words, and communication by intuition as a direct experience of the other person's feelings. Language was invented for presenting the material world, he argued. A direct impact, on the other hand, evokes feelings in us. It is not symbolic or semantic, and Bion called it non-sensuous perception. Whether "non-sensuous" is a good word or not, he was really referring to what we ordinarily call empathy. Implicitly, Bion linked this non-symbolic communication with projective identification.

Bion's interest was whether this kind of impact is a direct communication (or evocation) of that out-of-sight O, that psychoanalytic invariant which is the patient's experience. Perhaps it does not have to be tortuously transmitted through the patient's own awareness of their own state of mind, their choice of words, the analyst's receipt of those words, and what they can make of them. Can we cut through the world of appearances with a direct intuited sense of O? It is like when the infant is screaming and the mother is immediately filled with the baby's alarm and rushes to see what has happened.

These reflections on communication are a caesura in the development of Bion's thinking. From his Tavistock training onwards, he had been determined to treat psychoanalysis like a science, and had done all the work necessary to bring it into line with the scientific method. This he called a scientific vertex or point of view. Now he moved on and realised he might describe psychoanalysis as something else. No longer seeing psychoanalysis as a natural science, language needed to be foregone in favour of a non-symbolic, non-representing impact on others. In *Attention and Interpretation*, he was occupied with what else psychoanalysis could be. One of his patients in the late 1960s was Roland Harris, an amateur poet about whom his daughter wrote that he "was an analysand of Bion's until he left for California, and was probably influential in encouraging Bion's venture into fiction in the *Memoir*" (Harris Williams, 2010, p. 28, n10). Bion seemed ready in 1967 to consider that psychoanalysis might be more akin to aesthetics, more about evoking an impact than about formulating symbolic representations, descriptions, and abstract theories.

Summary

The dialogue in this part seems to revolve around a distinction between, on the one hand, the "as if" quality of symbolic representations that can be communicated in cognitive ways and, on the other, a kind of direct emotional impact which does not necessarily depend on semantic meanings. Bion stressed this distinction increasingly during his career, eventually adopting a notion of aesthetic evocation as constituting a different mode of communication between two minds than that offered by ordinary speech. Winnicott had already made this distinction early on with his focus on there being "no such thing as a baby".

In this dialogue, a significant engagement between Winnicott and Bion, taking place back in 1955, is addressed. Bion reported on part of his early work with a psychotic patient and the disintegration of ego-functions and their dispersal. The patient's lax inability to ring his mother was given an alternative meaning by Winnicott as an illustration of a deficient relationship with a primary object in the past recurring in the transference relationship. Due to Winnicott's different perspective, he wrote to Bion to say how he would have interpreted the patient's communication on the couch.

For both Winnicott and Bion there is a recognition of the infant's dependency, but a major difference is that in Winnicott's model the infant does not recognise it and mother's responsibility is to sustain the baby's "illusion of omnipotence" so long as this is gradually followed by a phase of disillusionment. In Bion's model the infant is much more exposed to awareness of its intolerable helplessness and dependence, and the mother's responsibility is, at first, the bodily care, which importantly communicates that she can understand the needs the infant cannot understand. The difference is that, on one hand, satisfaction allays the disintegrating effects of frustration and pain, and on the other, a response communicates an understanding of the frustration and thus a growth in the baby's own understanding of its experiences.

Winnicott's complex process by which the infant can be led out of the absolute dependency in five steps is significantly different from Bion's model of mental growth. Bion plots the process of an evolving sense of self coming into existence in relation to an external object. Winnicott's constant bodily care, with its mental satisfaction, contrasts with the constant repetition of the containing of intolerable experience by an *understanding* carer (Bion).

In Bion's work there is a turn towards recognising the importance of the mode of communication and the movement, especially in analysis, from direct evocation relying on the analyst's intuition towards a containment in mental representations or words. Winnicott was not always sure that verbal representation in the form of interpretation was the necessary

Table 4 Primary maternal preoccupation and making an impact

Winnicott	*Bion*
1. The core problem for the individual is dependency	1. Bion's focus returned to the method of listening
2. The mother is preoccupied with the infant because of her intense devoted identification	2. The patient's unconscious is the invariant "O"
3. A sense of continuity-of-being is set up at a deep level in healthy psychic beginnings	3. Bion came to consider intuition as a direct kind of non-symbolic communicative evocation in someone else
4. There is a five-stage sequence in early development involving object-relating from dependency	4. He sought to keep his own preconceptions as clear as possible from the work
5. Development starts with a merging with the object, followed by a gradual awareness of separateness and a destruction. Survival-of-the-object, and love	5. The analyst must avoid his own memory and desire in order to avoid interference with the patient's way of making sense
6. A process of object-relating to object usage occurs due to the psychic environment	

intervention, and he increasingly emphasised being as the process that would lead to knowing.

Dialogue

Jan Abram: The interests you indicate Bion moved on to in Chapter 8 have a strong resonance with Winnicott's work. I feel that now we're getting to the creative Bion who, I think, is beginning to "catch up" with Winnicott. As we indicated in Part III, it does seem that both authors were gaining momentum in their work from 1960 onwards, as if they felt free to express their own ideas without the concern of being criticised by Melanie Klein, or perhaps they were concerned not to hurt her if they disagreed with the concepts she held so dearly.

I was struck that you say at the beginning of your chapter that Bion was concerned to make sense of his own preconceptions without interfering with the patient's. This tallies with Winnicott, who said from the beginning of his work that it is the patient and only the patient who has the answers, and in his late work "The use of an object", he writes about how distressed he feels about making interpretations in the past that may well have interrupted the patients' processes. His emphasis in his chapters in *Playing and Reality* (Winnicott, 1971a) focus on "facilitating" and "waiting" for the patient's process. This is not so different from his earlier work, but this somehow took on new meaning for him at that time.

The paper in which Bion writes about abandoning memory and desire is, of course, quoted in countless ways, and I feel that many analysts idealise this notion. I don't know how different that specification is to free association and free-floating attention. In any case, I don't think it possible for an analyst to abandon memory or desire, but it is appropriate for the analyst to let go of a cognitive way of working with the patient and to focus on the notion of listening and being, which is what Winnicott advocated. I think that the aims of both authors for clinical analysis are quite close in this respect.

You say that Bion was focusing on his receptivity to the patient, and this is exactly what Winnicott was also interested in. In Chapter 7 I tried to explore the sequence of object-relating to object usage, which can only come about through the mother/analyst's receptivity. It is striking that Bion does not seem to have been interested in Winnicott's writings during that time. And while Bion is applying (or integrating) his Kantian philosophical point of view about perception, Winnicott is more interested in defining how the baby moves from apperception to perception in the trajectory from object-relating to object usage.

This is different from the way in which Bion spoke to his patient in the early 1950s, is it not? Especially the exchange he has in the paper on the psychotic and non-psychotic functioning. We had a dialogue about this during the IPA webinar, and you said that his aim was to change the patient's way of functioning. Winnicott would have eschewed this approach, and it seems you're saying that in his late work Bion had changed his mind about his earlier technique. Perhaps you could clarify this difference in Bion's technique.

Robert D. Hinshelwood: Technique is important for our dialogue. Bion's vivid memory from around 1930 of Wilfred Trotter's "unassumed listening" (Chapter 4) had struck a chord. Then, in his training in the 1940s, he would have attended lectures with Melanie Klein, and I gave a quote (in Chapter 4) from those recently published lectures to candidates: "If we are not bent on labelling our patients…only then, are we ready to learn step by step everything about the patient from himself" (Steiner, 2017, pp. 29–30).

Bion later echoed this: "In making his own model the analyst needs in such cases to be aware of and to lay bare the model used by the patient" (Bion, 1962a, p. 348). As we all know, since Freud it has been understood that it is the patient's unconscious which must lead us. But of course it is not so easy; the unconscious is by definition only known from clues.

You are quite right, Jan, that in the 1950s Bion moved away from using intuition, introspection, and countertransference and towards interpretation according to the theory of schizoid mechanisms. Subsequently, in the 1960s, there was another hiatus – and a movement back to introspective listening.

So, in the period when he was working with psychotic states (around 1950 to 1957), Bion interpreted according to a textbook of theories as much as introspection (he did in fact use introspection) of his own feelings about where he stood with his patients. For instance, in 1948, he had found countertransference more reliable than postulating the transference (see quote in Chapter 4). As you know, from around 1946 Bion was in supervision with Paula Heimann whose seminal 1949 paper on countertransference was published 1950. And Heimann's own training analyst in Berlin had been Theodor Reik, who published his *Listening with a Third Ear* in 1947. Clearly, together with his first analyst, John Rickman, Bion was among the analysts who from the 1930s were interested in countertransference.

So for Bion, later in the 1960s, it was a return home to his introspective, intuitive method of psychoanalytic sensitivity. Perhaps the difficulty of the psychosis work made the Klein group resort more to theory. One difficulty in following Bion is his change of focus from time to time. I once wrote a paper titled "Bion's nomadic journey", so titled because he was always on the move, zigzagging around. Another important change in the mid-1960s was his focus on the state of mind the analyst needs to cultivate. However, his prohibition on memory and desire is indeed somewhat crass. Any psychoanalyst is naïve to think that his unconscious dynamics could be so easily dealt with consciously. Nevertheless, he was investigating the state of mind he called a reverie, a condition in which one is open and receptive to the patient. He turned to Henri Poincaré on the "selected fact" in science, and to John Keats on "negative capability" in Shakespeare.

If I may say so, it would be helpful to spell out in more detail the means by which analyst and patient move through the five types of relations that you list in Chapter 7. What does the receptivity of the analyst actually do? For Bion it takes in the intolerable to survive the anxiety, modify it, and hand it back. What is the equivalent in Winnicott's method for taking the patient through each step?

J.A.: The emphasis on learning from the patient (a la Trotter) and Klein's citation is where the formulations of both of our protagonists come together, it seems to me. Doubtless, the majority of analysts would agree with this as a sine qua non of clinical practice. However, it is also true to say that the interpretation of "following the patient" will be different in each case, as it will depend on the gradual unfolding of the transference-countertransference matrix. This is why it is so important to listen to the patient and at the same time to listen to one's own affective responses while listening to the patient. Haydée Faimberg's work on "Listening to Listening" is key here (Faimberg, 1996). And as you point out, however experienced we are as analysts, we cannot be in control of what happens in our unconscious. This is something we all have to continually work on, which makes the practice of psychoanalysis both exciting and tiring at times. If we are not in touch with the psychic work we are obliged to go through with each patient, then we cannot be doing our job. I will come back to this point in answer to your question at the end of the last statement of the previous dialogue.

You convey quite regularly that Bion's trajectory in his psychoanalytic thinking was nomadic. I wonder how you understand why it was nomadic and why you use that term. By comparison, the evolution of Winnicott's thought is quite comprehensible when we examine how the concepts evolve in the three distinct periods of his particular journey (Abram, 2008). He has further thoughts, and elaborates consistently but does not change his mind much on the fundamental concepts he set out in his 1945 paper "Primitive emotional development", and he increasingly focuses on the power of the mother's state of mind and how it lives on in a variety of ways in each psyche from the beginning.

It was refreshing to see that you think Bion's "prohibition on memory and desire" was crass, even though you can see Bion's interest in saying that, its purpose was to home in on how the analyst needs to find a state of reverie. Where does he speak of survival, by the way? When you ask what is the equivalent of receptivity in Winnicott's method, I have to refer you (and the reader) back to Chapter 7, especially where I dissect Winnicott's five-step sequence, which defines the transition from object-relating to object usage. Let me give a brief comment here on how I understand the difference between Winnicott's technique (as seen in "The use of an object") and Bion's technique as you set it out in reference (especially) to his paper "The theory of thinking" (Bion, 1962b).

For Winnicott, there are two early psychic environments (you'll remember I referred to this thesis in Chapter 4 of our first book in this series). One psychic environment (that is, the mother's state of mind) is good enough, and the other is simply not good enough. In the good-enough scenario, the infant is not de facto in a state of intolerable anxiety at the beginning. On the contrary, due to the mother's state of absolute dedication to her newborn, the baby is only on a delicate brink of feeling overwhelmed, so it is certainly precarious, but because of the mother's holding capacities, the infant is protected from ever feeling flooded with intolerable anxieties. But if we examine what Winnicott means by the psychic environment that fails to protect the infant from falling forever, we see resonances with Klein's definition of the paranoid-schizoid position. Here is the difference, in my view, between Winnicott and Bion. For Winnicott, the paranoid-schizoid position constitutes the failure of the psychic environment (that is, a mother who cannot hold or contain her infant's primitive needs). What you describe, Bob, about Bion's ideas on receiving the infant's intolerable anxieties demonstrates for me that Bion, like you, (in Chapter 3 of our first book) followed Klein's formulation of the paranoid-schizoid position as a universal fact for all infants at the beginning of life.

Now, in the clinical situation, and following Freud's thoughts on regression, Winnicott recognises that the mother's failures will inevitably be re-evoked in the transference relationship and that this is where the analyst has to do something psychically that the mother has not been able to do. In an environment that is not good enough, the failure occurs at steps two, three, or four. If the five steps are not completed on a consistent level, then the infant is unable to reach the stage of the use of an object. Therefore, the work has to be achieved in the analysis, and this requires an enormous amount of psychic work on the part of the analyst – more so than the analysis of a patient who comes into the process already able to use the object (this isn't to say there is not further work to accomplish in the latter case).

R.D.H.: It is important, isn't it, that we note where Bion and Winnicott agree and don't find differences where there aren't any. There is a sense in which you are right that all analysts must have an intuitive sense of what the analysand is feeling and what their core unconscious phantasies are. So it is essential to acknowledge agreement. Moreover, Bion and Winnicott both learned most of their foundational psychoanalytic theories from Klein. Indeed, Winnicott was regarded as part of the group supporting Klein until the late 1940s; just about until Bion became a member of the society, when he, as it were, took over Winnicott's place, something it seems that neither of them could properly work through.

The difference in your last piece concerns two things, I think. One is the rejection of the paranoid-schizoid position by Winnicott, while

Bion more or less only uses the paranoid-schizoid position. Despite the contrasting emphases, both Winnicott and Bion would have agreed on the nature of the depressive position and their concern for the object as the core of growth and maturity. The second point is something I think haunted our previous work on Klein and Winnicott – that is, the actual experience of the infant that the adult (or child) still harbours.

Taking first the paranoid-schizoid position in the way it comes across in your account of Winnicott, once the infant has been failed and has tasted the sense of disintegration and loss of self (being), the sense of self can never be recovered except with a psychoanalyst. This is probably not really what you mean, and we might agree that probably no mother is completely perfect in being good enough, if I can put it like that. There must be times when a mother is less good than good enough (as well as times when she is more than good enough). So we have all been affected by that not-good-enough environment – some of us more than others. When the mother is less good, surely there must be means, or objects, other than psychoanalysis that can be used for recovery, no? If that is the case, then development is a fluctuating process of moving nearer and then further away from that catastrophic experience. My guess is that Winnicott's "fear of breakdown" might be the equivalent to what Klein called a fear of survival and Bion a fear of death. But if there is a fluctuating process, then that is exactly what Bion accepted from Klein. All through life we go in and out of paranoid-schizoid states of mind. It would not be possible to conscript men into an army unless they were able to enter a state of mind dominated by a determination to exterminate those other soldiers who are believed to be determined to exterminate them. There is, in Bion's view, a constant movement from violently hating a dangerous other to a concern for the other who one wished to destroy and back again. In other words, (in your terms) the two different external environments alternate. As one of my teachers many years ago described it, there is a move from fighting against something to fighting for something. This may need more discussion, perhaps.

The second point was what I experience as the need for a more "experience-near" descriptions of the analytic sessions, through the five stages you define. I need to get into the feeling states. As you seem to suggest, there is no experience of hatred, destruction, and murder in normal development. It raises the question: What are the experiences an infant does go through? With the good-enough environment, is it just love or nothing, one or the other? I think this is probably not quite your position. Certainly, Winnicott talks of 18 reasons for hate in the countertransference, doesn't he? And he is sure all mothers hate their babies at times. In which of the stages does the experience of hate have to be struggled with? How does the baby deal with it? How does the mother/carer deal with it and help the infant to evolve towards a realistic fight *for* something? I am asking not just for a description of the kinds of relations in the five stages but for an evocation of the both participants' feelings in the struggles and anxieties of each stage. For instance, at what point does the infant know there is an external separate object, and what does it feel like (I suspect it is complete impotence and dependent helplessness, all of a sudden)? And what does mother feel? A wrenching loss, an amputation, perhaps?

J.A.: Yes, Bob, it is important to distinguish between areas of agreement and disagreement. Both of our protagonists were very influenced by Melanie Klein, but perhaps Bion more than Winnicott because he was in analysis with her. Perhaps this meant that Winnicott could keep a distance, although he clearly had a powerful transference towards her. I often think that there was something about Klein's personal depression that might have resonated for Winnicott because of his experience with his own mother, who was evidently depressed.

I don't think I see Bion as "taking over Winnicott's place", as you put it. I'm reminded of something Juliet Mitchell said many years ago at a Winnicott study day at Jesus College, Cambridge, that Bion was the legitimate son of Klein while Winnicott was her illegitimate son. I think Bion was fostered by Klein and her followers in a way that Winnicott was most definitely not. And we know that Bion, before he went to California, was very active in the Melanie Klein Trust. Winnicott became President of the British Psychoanalytic Society on two occasions (like his father, who had been the mayor of Plymouth on two occasions).

I was struck by what you said about Bion seeming to exclusively use the paranoid-schizoid position in his work. That makes sense suddenly. It is in contrast to Winnicott's focus on delineating aspects of health in order to recognise how psychopathology comes about: in his theory it is always because of the deficiency of the psychic environment.

The issue of what is good enough and not good enough is what Winnicott was trying to define throughout most of his life's work. But when you say that the infant has a "sense of disintegration and loss of self that can never be recovered except with a psychoanalyst", I think it important to clarify what I was attempting to say.

So, what is not good enough at the very start, when the infant is just a newborn, will be catastrophic. This is a picture of extreme trauma to the infant's psyche. Therefore, there is no disintegration because there has not yet been time for the infant to start to integrate. Also, there is no loss of self because the infant does not yet have an evolved self. There is only environmental failure, and the outcome is infantile trauma, which is at the root of psychosis. In fact, this is the definition of madness.

Later you say that I said there is "no experience of hatred, destruction, and murder in normal development". But that is not the picture in Winnicott's paradigm. What I was wishing to convey is that at the very start of life the infant is not capable of feeling murderous hate because these affects, along with love, envy, and sadism, have not yet developed. Hate and envy are affects that evolve in the infantile psyche as a result of the early environment. These affects will, of course, evolve in normal development, but they will be extreme when the infant has not had a good-enough start.

There are certainly struggles at the start of life for the baby. Winnicott writes about the precariousness of these early stages which the mother is able to protect the baby from so that they do not psychically fall. If the mother "Fails" at these earliest stages (note the upper case "F" to indicate gross impingement on the psyche resulting in psychic trauma), then the baby will fall and suffer primitive agony. The mother's function to begin with is to prevent that from happening, and that is the definition of "good enough". The baby is fortunate due to the mother's strong ego protection.

Because Winnicott's focus is on a gradual development, little by little, as the infant starts to experience the externality of the object (distinguishing Me from Not-Me), there is no such thing as "complete impotence and dependent helplessness", as you suggest, because the process of emotional development is never "complete". This is avoided because of the mother's attunement. Therefore, because of her ability to take each step one at a time, the extreme anxieties are avoided, which means they never flood the psyche of both the mother and her baby.

R.D.H.: I think it is really helpful to try to convey (however impossible it is to do so completely) the actual experience of a baby in these early steps. And I would like to get *into* those experiences more. You convey that there are no ordinary feelings of love, hate, and so on. So what is the experience of unintegration? My associations go back to Glover and Brierley and their descriptions of ego-nuclei and a sort of bits-and-pieces kind of experience. And the sense of falling into "primitive agony" is what Glover and Brierley might call "bursting", is that right? But how did Winnicott convey the actual experience of primitive agony so that one could recognise it in one's patient. They are not going to say, "I've got a primitive agony"; so what manifestation makes us say, "Oh good heavens – he's in primitive agony".

However, since we are concerned with Bion, rather than Klein, we can say, I think, that Bion really was not interested in the early infant as a relevant conception at all. He referred always to the here-and-now experience, what he called "realisations" because they are real for the people present. He came to psychoanalysis via group dynamics. And those dynamics of the group had no infantile beginning. He quickly moved to working with and researching psychotic states, where the primitive was there in front of him, not "back there and then". He could construct his impression of primitiveness as he was caught up in the dynamics now. It is vivid in Bion's description, for instance:

> When the patient glanced at me he was taking a part of me into him. It was taken into his eyes, as I later interpreted his thought to him, as if his eyes could suck something out of me. This was then removed from me, before I sat down, and expelled, again through his eyes, so that it was deposited in the right-hand corner of the room where he could keep it under observation while he was lying on the couch. The expulsion took a moment or two to complete.
>
> (Bion, 1958, pp. 113–114)

Here Bion is trying to discover a way of talking about the experience of a hallucinating state of mind,in which perceptions are experienced in very concrete ways. Whatever one thinks of his actual description of the experience, he was trying to get inside that experience. Many have doubted whether this is really the patient's experience, as opposed to being merely a construction of Bion's, and it has often been recognised that there may be a similarity between this kind of construction and his experience of the battlefield, where bits of shrapnel were flying everywhere. One of those doubters of his descriptions was Bion himself, who eventually despaired of giving an accurate account: "I do not regard any narrative purporting to be a report of fact, either of what the patient said or of what I said, as worth consideration as a 'factual account' of what happened" (Bion, 1967, p. 53). And from that point on he evolved a distinction between the kind of description just given – that of a more objective kind – and something more like feeling it in the gut, which defies verbal description. So what is necessary is an evocation, non-verbal, non-symbolic, which just constitutes a direct hit on the other person. He called this "an evolutionary change of perspective" (Bion, 1967, p. 1), and he tried to capture it in this way (as previously noted):

> The point that demonstrates the divergence most clearly is that the physician is dependent on realisation of sensuous experience in contrast with the psycho-analyst whose dependence is on experience that is not sensuous. The physician can see and touch and smell. The realisations with which a psycho-analyst deals cannot be seen or touched; anxiety has no shape or colour, smell or sound. For convenience, I propose to use the term "intuit" as a parallel in the psychoanalyst's domain to the physician's use of "see", "touch", "smell", and "hear".
>
> (Bion, 1970, p. 7)

I don't know if Winnicott made any comparable distinction between objective observation and subjective intuition. If not, why not? And why was Bion so exercised by it? Is the answer that he was an Edwardian gentleman, originating in that Victorian stiff-upper-lip tradition of the British Raj, trying to unstiffen his experiences? For whatever reason, Bion was driven to investigate this alternative domain, where apprehension or apperception of his patients' experience occurs without interference. And interference includes remembering the patient from yesterday and the intrusion of giving in to hopes of cure and so forth. This was radical, and in the 1970s he turned over in his mind whether psychoanalysis was a scientific enterprise at all, whether it had to move away from objective observation and theoretical inferencing. Indeed, he went so far as to say that, quite possibly, psychoanalysis is an aesthetic enterprise, based on evocation rather than observation. To this end, he wrote three novels (Bion, 1975, 1977, 1979) aimed at putting aside common sense and reason and trying to evoke inspiration and a flow of dreamlike consciousness. In my view, he flirted with surrealism. And surrealism had grown out of just this inspirational, dreamlike state that psychoanalysis points to. Moreover, Bion had been in France (Poitiers) in the 1920s, when French surrealism was at its peak.

I think Winnicott made no comment on Bion's attempt to take a radical direction in the radical 1970s, did he? What might he have thought of the possibility of relinquishing his objectivity about mother-baby relations and replacing it with that intuitive subjectivity of his gut reactions in the analytic session? The debate between them would, it seems, have been about the very nature of psychoanalysis itself. I have often had an impression in our discussions that Winnicott was somewhat blind to the distinction between objective observation and subjective experiencing. Marjorie Brierley (1937) says Bion was interested in "rapport", and maybe it would help if we could distinguish rapport from verbal communication.

J.A.: I found your last paragraph provocative, Bob, and I wondered why I reacted like this. Let me start by saying a word about the analytic culture I was brought up in (that of psychotherapy and psychoanalysis since the early 1980s in London). You were already an analyst in that culture and made several groundbreaking contributions. You set up the *British Journal of Psychotherapy*, which was a major success and is still going strong. And you published your dictionary on Klein's thought in 1989, which was inspirational for many and certainly inspired me, among other influences like Laplanche and Pontalis, to write *The Language of Winnicott* (Abram, 2007).

Don't you remember the general perspective at that time, which still prevails to some extent today, that Winnicott worked sensitively and was the most intuitive of all psychoanalysts of the twentieth century? This was in contrast to a view that Kleinians, because of their preoccupation with aggression, do not protect the patient from interpretations which "go for the jugular". Added to this was the view that Winnicott was like a teddy bear who encouraged his patients to regress and broke analytic boundaries while Klein and her followers were correctly following the patients' unconscious, especially the worst aspects of the unconscious (that is, hate, sadism, and envy). Winnicott and the Independents were empathic and attuned to their patients while Klein, Bion, Segal, and Joseph were correctly showing their patients how envy and hate caused them to suffer. Winnicott did not interpret enough and the Kleinians interpreted too much so that there was no analytic space for reflection and free association, I'm aware what I've just written above are clichés; nevertheless, many analysts still maintain these perspectives from each clinical paradigm. We tried to address the "myths" about each other's work in our first book of this series (Abram and Hinshelwood, 2018).

So when you asked what Winnicott "might have thought of the possibility of relinquishing his objectivity about mother-baby relations and replacing it with that intuitive subjectivity of his gut reactions in the analytic session" and then stated that he was "somewhat blind to the distinction between objective observation and subjective experiencing", I had a visceral reaction and felt shocked by your view of Winnicott as a clinician. But in the wake of this I am realising that I don't seem to have managed to convey to you, in the context of the first book and now coming to the final part of this book, that for me and many who follow Winnicott's work all over the world, what makes his clinical innovations so meaningful is related to his extraordinary clinical acumen. How could he possibly have formulated all his psychoanalytic advances without being attuned to his analytic clinical work with his patients? I know I am repeating myself, but I feel it needs to be said again that for Winnicott, being in contact with his own infantile layers helped him appreciate the adult patient on the couch *more* than working with infants. I think Winnicott was among the analysts who exemplified a capacity for rapport, to continue using Marjorie Brierley's term (Brierley, 1937).

Our common aim in this book is to eschew clichéd perspectives. It is too easy to say that Winnicott was sensitive and Klein, and therefore Bion, was not. Actually, I think it is clear that all three were working out ways of facilitating their patients.

Like you, Bob, I am also very interested in Marjorie Brierley's work (compare Abram, 2022) and have suggested that her work anticipates the concept of countertransference. I think you are right that it will help if we can "distinguish rapport from verbal communication", and I think this takes us organically into the final part of this book, where we intend to discuss the concepts of countertransference and technique. I hope to be able to elaborate on the questions you are asking about "objective observation and subjective intuition".

R.D.H.: I think you express very perceptively a lot of the mythology that exists (and has existed since the Controversial Discussions) about different schools of analysts. Indeed, one could identify a school of psychoanalysts not only by the metapsychology they accept but by the misconceptions they have of other schools. And we do have to be careful of each other's sensitivities when "projecting" views into their metapsychology. It is tempting to respond on the basis of Kleinian sensitivity to the description of her "going for the jugular" or "closing off space for reflection", and so on. Indeed, as you say, our books are intended to set aside such myths. And I am sorry if I seem to have belittled Winnicott's clinical intuition.

Maybe I need to clarify just a little, at risk of clumsily putting my foot into it further. I do actually think that Winnicott's formulations are limited, just as Bion's are. Their work is now more than half a century old, and though psychoanalysis is a slowly advancing discipline, it has developed beyond the work of Bion or Winnicott. We do have a responsibility to try to understand each other as accurately as possible, but even more so, we have a responsibility to understand our patients. In Chapter 4 I quoted Klein on how we must "learn step by step everything about the patient from himself". It is part of a longer quote indicating how we must put aside theory and generalisations that we have already generated. So when Winnicott used his immense experience as a paediatrician to observe and make generalisations about what a baby does with a spatula, it was different from his intuition in a clinical session when he found himself thinking he was mad because he saw his middle-aged male patient as a young woman. The first is an objective set of perceptions used to create a theory, or at least a general model. The second is an insight coming from his own internal observation of his feelings and reactions in a specific moment with a specific patient.

Maybe Winnicott would not have seen a difference between those two mental attitudes and processes, although I suspect he would have seen such a difference. For Bion, that difference was something the significance of which grew progressively throughout his career until it reached an overriding importance in his clinical work. The need to set aside objective and generalised knowledge became a clinical priority in his work with patients (and indeed in debate with psychoanalytic colleagues). He even thought that anything he had already learned about a particular patient should be set aside in the following session – in each session one should set one's mind as if seeing a completely new patient. For this, some people have roundly criticised him. However, he became more and more convinced that knowledge clogs up the mind, rendering the analyst less receptive to continued learning about and from the patient.

And thus to Part V…

J.A.: Yes, Bob – let's go now on to our fifth and final part of this book. Because it is in that part that we will home in on the specific techniques of our protagonists and see how they compare.

But before that, I do feel obliged to say something about the distinction you make between Winnicott's observations of infants when he was working as a paediatrician and his insights based on countertransference affects in the session with patients in analysis. While I think there are some differences to be teased out, since being a child doctor and being an analyst are different de facto, I think the bedrock of his observations was his abiding experience of being a patient in analysis. In other words, his observations emanated from his profound insights related to an ongoing contact with the infantile depths of his personality. As I've quoted above, he was very clear that he could not see the newborn as a human being until he had completed five years of his personal analysis, which gave him insights into the infantile layer of his psyche. This fundamental experience of being in high-frequency analysis for many years or decades cannot be bypassed or overlooked (not that I am saying you are doing so).

I am sure that my own experience, more than twenty years in total, of two different analyses with two different analysts informs not only how I am in the consulting room with my patients but also how I write, how I think, and how I live. Psychoanalysis, for me, is a way of life beyond working and practising as a psychoanalyst. And this is an interesting angle from which to examine what you said above about "objective observation and subjective intuition". I think these distinctions are the sine qua non of psychoanalytic practice, and they are the focus of the next part of this book.

PART V

CLINICAL APPROACH

These final chapters address the concepts of countertransference and technique. Convergences and divergences are examined to highlight fundamental differences. The authors' clinical examples show how Winnicott and Bion's final formulations determined their clinical approach. Winnicott's focus was on the mother's early role in the transference and, Bion's focus was on the here and now in the transference.

DOI: 10.4324/9781003382409-14

CHAPTER NINE

"A sample of the original failure"

Jan Abram

Winnicott's approach to analytic technique was fundamentally based on the way in which he had internalised the experience of analysis with both James Strachey (1923–1933) and Joan Riviere (1934–1944). Each analysis had been conducted at a frequency of five sessions weekly.

In Winnicott's obituary for James Strachey, he emphasised that Strachey had identified a process, based on his analysis with Freud, that develops in the patient such that "what transpires cannot be produced but it can be made use of". His experience of analysis with Strachey, Winnicott wrote, "has made me suspicious of descriptions of interpretative work…which give credit to the interpretations for all that happens, as if the process in the patient had got lost sight of" (Winnicott, 1969b). In this same obituary of 1967, Winnicott highlights that Strachey's main contribution, apart from his being general editor of Freud's *Complete Works*, was to make explicit "the principle of economic interpretation… at the point of urgency, accurately timed, gathering together the material presented by the patient and clearly dealing with a sample of transference neurosis" (Winnicott, 1969b).

In the first book of this series I emphasised in Chapter 10 how Winnicott's notion of the holding environment, also indicated in this book, was an essential component in making it possible for the analyst to

DOI: 10.4324/9781003382409-15

offer a mutative interpretation. This is tied in with the patient's capacity to receive the interpretation and to make meaning of it.

Notably, when Winnicott wrote this obituary he was at the point of writing his well-known paper "The use of an object", in which he emphasises how the analyst should wait for the patient to make their own interpretation. Elsewhere, he emphasised that interpretation can be like indoctrination if not given in the "ripeness of time" (Winnicott, 1971a).

In a letter written to Bion after the latter had given his paper "The differentiation of the psychotic and non psychotic personalities", Winnicott wanted to show Bion how he would have interpreted to Bion's patient. Bion's interpretations to the patient addressed the psychotic part of the personality, which uses splitting/projective identification "as a substitute for repression". Repression is the mechanism employed by the non-psychotic personality. Bion infers that for all individuals there exists a psychotic and non-psychotic part of each personality. This formulation emerges out of his opinion, following Klein, that the paranoid-schizoid position is universal at the beginning of life. It seems to follow from this that the baby is psychotic at the beginning. This is one of the basic assumptions underlying his theory.

In contrast to Bion's Kleinian view, Winnicott's perspective on the development of the psyche was that the impact of the psychic environment had to be taken into account. Therefore, for Winnicott, psychosis constituted an "environmental deficiency disease" arising out of the early failures of the psychic environment. In Winnicott's theory of trauma, psychosis is distinct from psychotic defences (Winnicott, 1960; Abram, 2021). In the course of any given analysis, therefore, the patient will inevitably regress in the transference to the layer on which the original maternal failure will be reached.

This is Winnicott's point when he wrote to Bion on 7 October 1955, after Bion had presented his paper at a Scientific Meeting of the British Psychoanalytical Society. In this excerpt Winnicott describes to Bion how he would have interpreted to the patient.

To begin with, he explains that if a patient of his lay on the couch moving and, as Bion describes, then said he should have phoned his mother, he (Winnicott) would know he was talking about an incapacity to communicate. Following this observation, Winnicott would then go on to say to the patient:

> A mother properly oriented to her baby would know from your movements what you need. There would be a communication because

> of this knowledge which belongs to her devotion and she would do something which would show that the communication had taken place. I am not sensitive enough or oriented in that way to be able to act well enough and therefore I in this present analytic situation fall into the category of the mother who failed to make communication possible. In the present relationship therefore, there is given a sample of the original failure from the environment which contributed to your difficulty in communication.
>
> (Winnicott, 1955 in Rodman, 1987)

Winnicott says that he felt Bion was talking about the environment by bringing this clinical material, which showed that the patient lacked an ordinary capacity to communicate because his mother had failed in her original task at the very beginning (Winnicott, 1955). Winnicott was clear that the presented clinical material "screamed out for an interpretation about communication". Winnicott's proposed interpretation, I have suggested, constitutes what Freud called a "construction", which is when the analyst "lays before the subject of the analysis a piece of his early history that he has forgotten" (Freud, 1937, p. 261). Paradoxically, in the context of the analytic situation, by making this construction the analyst is able to do something the original object could not; that is, receive the communication that the early mother had failed to receive. Now, in the present tense of the analytic situation, the "sample of the original failure" is relived in the transference. In his letter to Bion, Winnicott strongly implied that Bion's technique was in danger of violating the patient's unconscious communication by "taking it in abstract", which, he wrote, is "always a dangerous thing to do" (Winnicott, 1955).

Psychosis and psychotic states originate in ruptures in the continuity-of-being. The "fear of breakdown" in the future is based on the breakdown that has already occurred (in early psychic development) before the infant could discern Me from Not-Me (compare Abram, 2013, pp 205–212).

Winnicott's proposed construction speaks to the infantile level in the adult on the couch who has been traumatised. This amounts to a rupture in the continuity-of-being. The analytic situation replicates the holding environment for all patients, but for the psychotic, Winnicott pointed out, *"the couch IS the analyst's lap or womb, and the warmth IS the live warmth of the analyst's body"*(Winnicott, 1947). Talking to a patient as if they are a neurotic and therefore understand transference as an illusion (because they are able to play with it) is quite different from how the analyst speaks to a patient who may be experiencing a psychotic transference. An abstract interpretation may reinforce the delusional transference. I think this is what Winnicott implied in his letter to Bion.

The importance of the oedipal layer and the primal scene in clinical psychoanalysis is not negated in Winnicott's work on the early parent-infant relationship. On the contrary, his work amplifies and adds to the classical Freudian paradigm by showing that the infantile area at the very beginning cannot be separated from the quality of the mother's holding at the start. The father will only take his position as a significant third *if* the mother has retained him in her mind so that the infant's paternal integrate has evolved into a paternal imago (Abram, 2022, pp. 132–144).

The analyst does not imitate the mother of the early stages. Rather, through the polyphony of her affective responses, she follows the "Ariadne thread" of the transference dynamics (Brierley, 1936). Session by session, day by day, week by week, year by year, she gathers together her analysand's constructions of their psychic history. The analytic holding, emulating the mother's holding, constitutes both the frame and process of the treatment. But for me, the key to a successful holding is the psychic *survival-of-the-object* proposed by Winnicott in his late work (1969a). In the clinical situation it will be the analyst's capacity to live through a multitude of ineffable affects and experiences that emerge not only from the patient's infantile layer of experience but from variable layers of developmental moments. This consistent work will gradually offer the analysand a route to a new organisation of temporality in which the original failures can have an opportunity to be worked through.

CHAPTER TEN

Content and process

R.D. Hinshelwood

Bion's publications after the mid-60s became rare. He was thinking about transformations from learning to something he called "growth". The concept of growth does not emerge very clearly, but it would seem to be that more organic, unsettled state of direct impact described in Chapter 8. One can see the method of approach he developed in his seminars, which he conducted on three continents from the mid-60s onwards. His style was provocative and challenging, and perhaps he felt there was more chance of a direct experience coming alive than in a deadening report of a session.

Bion had escaped the tight conformity of the British Psychoanalytical Society in 1968. In California there was the freedom to explore new ideas, however weird. Bion's development was not in the direction of weirdness. There are only few published works from this period. Entries in his notebook (Bion, 1992) become sparse and brief, but he wrote three volumes of autobiography (published posthumously). His main published work before his death in 1979 was a trilogy of novels with the overall title *Memoir of the Future*.

DOI: 10.4324/9781003382409-16

Aesthetic "truth"

It appears his interest in exploring psychoanalysis as an aesthetic rather than a scientific practice persisted through the 1970s, when he considered the nature of lying. Normally a lie covers some unpalatable truth; it is the opposite of truth. Nevertheless, when Virginia Woolf wrote *Mrs. Dalloway*, she did not write a "true story". Strictly speaking it is untrue, but it has an artistic truth. Yet, at the moment when the character Septimus Smith leans out over the windowsill and falls to his death, there is a powerful reaction in the reader. His craziness (perhaps a result of PTSD) makes his suicide shocking, despairing, and very painful. It has an impact on the reader, and is true for them. In his work on lies, Bion's intention was to explore this communication of truth. Perhaps it motivated his autobiographical writing, which shocks as much as it describes. He made a distinction between having an impact and communicating a pregnant meaning, which came to a head in this last period of Bion's life.

When Bion presented an impossible case in his seminars in Los Angeles in 1967 and again in 1968 in Buenos Aires (Aguayo and Malin, 2013; Aguayo, de Cortinas, and Regczkey, 2017), he may have been attempting to have an impact. The woman he described certainly did. She conducted the session in a scream or worse. Bion attempted to convey "the full, the blast of [this] experience" (Bion, 1967, p. 85), which left him unable to know what he was thinking, let alone what the patient was. Bion seems to have been challenging his audience to contemplate this impact and how it felt, to step out of the realm of professional, measured debate. Even just reading the transcript of the seminar, one is filled with unmanageable reactions. In his previous seminars, Bion at times seemed to be trying to convey the impact of unprocessed beta-elements (see Chapter 6), which are antithetical to thoughts.

Symbol-interpretation or process-interpretation

This intense involvement in the impact exemplifies (although it did not originate) a clinical approach that had diverged from Freud many years before. Interpretation takes account of a narrative, a process played out between the two individuals. This is different from the interpretation of dream symbols. Symbols are simply interpreted as that which they are intended to hide. Instead of dream interpretation, Bion emphasised the narrative process involving both analysand and analyst.

Moreover, the attempt to grasp the narrative originates in the analyst's focus on the role he is induced to play out with the patient. Bion had always stressed what he learned from introspection to decide the most likely role that seemed to be required of him in the narrative.

This intuitive introspection regarding narrative remains a strong tradition today, as seen in the work of Betty Joseph (1989) and her colleagues including Steiner (2000) and Feldman (2007). Joseph, for instance, described the narrative meaning of the session as an enactment or a potential one; for instance:

> Patient A begins a session by telling me that once again he has been extremely nasty with his wife on the previous night and he enumerates a series of apparently unkind, intolerant things that he has done and his wife's responses. It sounds from this that he might be experiencing what we could call superego anxiety – guilt about what he has done and a desire to get the analyst to understand and explain the reasons for his behaviour. Or he might be speaking about his anxiety about his wife and her ruthlessness and the bad state of the marriage; i.e. is it depression, sorrow and guilt that he is talking about, or persecution and hatred? Or is he telling me about the failure of my work, that once again he has had one of these rows? Or is it to be understood as an acting out from the relationship with the analyst?
>
> (Joseph, 1978, p. 223)

There are a number of narratives that the analyst hears, and some include the analyst herself. And then one of them clicks in some way – as she says:

> Actually, from my sense of what was going on, from the way that the patient was talking and the atmosphere that was being created in the session, it seemed to me that the most important aspect was the patient's attempt to involve me in a kind of verbal sadomasochistic beating of himself. I was being invited to join in by being interpretatively condemning or critical.
>
> (Joseph, 1978, p. 223)

Joseph's introspective method follows Bion's respect for intuiting the selected fact that evolves in the mind, as described by Poincaré (2011).

The tradition of interpreting unconscious narratives in the session remains a key element derived from the idea of continuous unconscious phantasy in the deeper layers of the unconscious mind. The deepest of those phantasies can be discerned in the narratives accepted, enacted, and then discovered by introspection via the roles unconsciously required of the analyst.

Bion's trajectory, though erratic in a theoretical sense as he found himself influenced by his reading (much of it outside of the psychoanalytic literature), tended to be in a consistent direction clinically. The lie is the careful manipulation of ideas, symbols, and memories. The truth of a session is the impact. That impact was something that Bion seemed to have remained true to even before he had started training as a psychoanalyst.

The psychoanalytic session is less important in terms of the content of meaning, and must be addressed in terms of process. And in particular, one needs to follow what one mind *does* to the other. This action on another mind is not just the transference but the reaction to the analyst's intervention. Let us return to a session Bion reported in the early years of his psychoanalytic work, the session referred to in Jan's Chapter 9. We can see how Bion found a way of *doing* something with the material, rather than simply interpreting content from the past or present. Let me give a little of the reported material, which may make Jan's comments clearer in relation to what Bion was doing. To present Bion's material is a little difficult, as he interpolates long passages of reflection and speculation, so the following is pared back to simplify the dialogue between the patient and analyst:

He had arrived 15 minutes late:

PATIENT: I don't suppose I shall do anything today. I ought to have rung up my mother.

[Pause]

PT: No; I thought it would be like this.

[PROLONGED PAUSE]

PT: Nothing but filthy things and smells, I think I've lost my sight.

[25 minutes had passed]

ANALYST: I told him that these filthy things and smells were what he felt he had made me do, and that he felt he had compelled me to defecate them out, including the sight he had put in to me.

[The patient jerked convulsively and I saw him cautiously scanning what seemed to be the air around him]

AN: I said he felt surrounded by bad and smelly bits of himself including his eyes which he felt he had expelled from his anus.

PT: I can't see.

AN: I then told him he felt he had lost his sight and his ability to talk to his mother, or to me, when he had got rid of these abilities so as to avoid pain.

PT: My head is splitting; may be my dark glasses.

AN: Your sight has come back into you but splits your head; you feel it is very bad sight because of what you have done to it.
PT: [Moving in pain as if protecting his back passage] Nothing.
AN: It seemed to be your back passage.
PT: Moral strictures.
AN: I told him that his sight, the dark glasses, were felt as a conscience that punished him, partly for getting rid of them to avoid pain, partly because he had used them to spy on me, and on his parents.
PT: The week-end; don't know if I can last it.

This is the important moment. After the interpretation, the patient began to experience an aspect of reality, a painful reality.

AN: You feel that you have to be able to get on without me. But to do that you feel you need to be able to see what happens around you, and even to be able to contact me; to be able to contact me at a distance, as you do your mother when you ring her up; so you tried to get your ability to see and talk back again from me.
PT: Brilliant interpretation. [With a sudden convulsion] O God!
AN: You feel you can see and understand now, but what you see is so brilliant that it causes intense pain.
PT: [Clenching his fists and showing much tension and anxiety] I hate you.
AN: When you see, what you see – the week-end break and the things you use darkness to spy on – fills you with hate of me and admiration.

(Bion, 1957, pp. 103–107)

Bion did something important. His interpretation brought together fragments that seemed displaced from one another:

- his sight
- the dark glasses
- his conscience in pain, and
- spying on the analyst and his parents

The narrative was that bringing back bits of material and putting them together momentarily restored the reality of the weekend; but in effect it restored his reality principle from its fragments . Bion enacted the bringing together. The response to the interpretation, Bion claimed, showed his interpretative re-integration of bits to be correct.

I want to emphasise that Bion really did think that the parts of the ego could very concretely be separated off and located in another person's mind, or elsewhere. And as in the excerpt above, interpretation is aimed at gathering the bits and pieces together again. However, this gathering of the patient's mind into a whole results in the tension and anxiety which was the cause of the splitting up of the functions. But restoring the functions and facing the head-splitting pain now occurs in the context of analysis, where someone else is able to understand. This was one of the origins of Bion's idea of containing, for the patient, the functions and the understanding which otherwise destroy the mind.

Summary

In this part a significant engagement between Winnicott and Bion is addressed. Debate between different schools was uncommon in the British Psychoanalytic Society after the Controversial Discussions in the 1940s. Nevertheless, judging by Winnicott's letters, he did not disregard Bion's work, and his comments reveal a difference in technique when working through the psychotic phase of the patient's analysis.

In describing the nature, use, and effect of interpretations, more divergence may become apparent. In these chapters in Part V, both Winnicott and Bion were shown to be concerned about the accuracy of interpretations. Winnicott questioned the value of only giving interpretations as, he says, they can be merely the analyst's theoretical views rather than constituting a real understanding of the patients' experiences. Bion emphasised a similar point in the course of doubting the capacity of analysts to accurately convey clinical material in discussions with each other. Bion regarded a true report of a session as requiring the representation of the analyst's direct experience at the time. Bion argued that the analyst had to attempt to receive those direct emotional communications and needed to supplant memory and desire with the experience of the moment. Winnicott, aware of those potential distortions, turned to other possible interventions, and held the view that it is better to wait for the patient to arrive at their own interpretation rather than accept the analyst's.

Bion regarded the most valid interpretations as those which grasped the narrative process going on in the session between analyst and patient in the moment. The analyst has to assess, introspectively, the role assigned to them in that context. This, he thought, represented a negotiation of an unconscious phantasy active in the present moment for the patient. Words are just as likely to be untruthful manipulations as they are to be true renderings of unconscious material. Winnicott regarded verbal material as a playing out of a long-forgotten trauma with a deficient early psychic environment/mother.

Both Winnicott and Bion agreed that interpreting to people in a psychotic state requires special attention. Winnicott regarded the transference as an unconscious communication of a psychic trauma that had not yet been received by the object. Rather differently, Bion, agreeing with the concreteness of the experience for someone in a psychotic state, moved from interpreting the experience to interpreting how the ego had lost the functions needed to recognise the true reality. He focused on the fragmentation itself.

One final difference between our two protagonists was in their consideration of who one speaks to when making an interpretation. Winnicott spoke to the early traumatised infant in the patient. In contrast, Bion, recognising perhaps that the infant (or in Bion's terms, the psychotic part of the patient) cannot use words, addresses the mature self with the intended consequence that words strengthen those functions in the more mature self which allow it to gain some dominance over the psychotic

Table 5 Failure and process

Winnicott	*Bion*
1. Interpretative work of the analyst can mistakenly take priority over processes in the patient	1. Clinical reporting needs to be a direct experience
2. Transference is an aspect of the truth about how the patient experienced the early psychic environment	2. Lies are the manipulation of words but truth is the emotional impact
3. Original failures are worked through by addressing ineffable affects	3. Narratives play out as here-and-now unconscious phantasies
4. We wait for the patient to reach their own interpretation	4. Aesthetic evocation is a form of truth
5. The transference to a failing analyst is common	5. When the narrative is fragmentation, interpretation brings fragments together.
6. Analyst emulates mother's holding at the bodily and psychic levels	6. Introspective analysis of the role played in a session (= countertransference) is primary
7. The analytic environment offers psychic *survival-of-the-object* of ruthless/destructive needs	7. Interpretations become a part of the transference narrative
8. Psychotic transference could be associated with trauma and treated by an object who survives instead of not surviving	8. Interpretation of a narrative played out in a session is not a static interpretation of a symbol

self. Possibly identifying the problem of speaking to the non-verbal infant, Winnicott recognised that when a patient regresses to an infantile level, interpretation does not work. What is required is more a focus on the actual context in the room of the analyst; the couch, the warmth, the soothing sounds, and so on.

Dialogue

Jan Abram: I was very struck, Bob, that Bion's publications in the mid 1960s were rare. But, as you show, he was continuing to develop his ideas, particularly on clinical work. But it reminded me about Winnicott's development during the same period. Elsewhere (Abram, 2008), I referred to his final eleven years, 1960–1971, as being associated with more of a philosophical inquiry; that is, what is it that makes life worth living? He was also preoccupied with the sense of feeling real. Due to being in continuous demand to speak, he wrote over one hundred articles on child development and at least 70 psychoanalytic papers. In the analytic relationship he stresses the need for the analyst to wait and to pay attention to the analysand's pace and capacity to grow. He advanced the technique of free association by identifying how, in the ordinary exchange between analyst and analysand, it is the capacity for the analytic pair to be engaged in play which facilitates the patient's contacting the self. I had previously pointed out that Bollas, following Winnicott, argues that the technique of free association has been undermined in contemporary psychoanalysis through an overuse of "here and now" transference interventions (Bollas, 2002; 2007). In this dialogue at the end of our book, we now have an opportunity to scrutinise the distinctions between Bion's technique of here-and-now transference interpretations and Winnicott's way of monitoring the patient's capacity to play in the analytic frame.

I was also struck that Bion was focusing more on the sense of aliveness in reported sessions. This seems to me to be parallel with Winnicott's quest for aliveness, years previously, when he criticised a "towing of the party line" in scientific discussions in the wake of the conclusions of the Controversial Discussions.

As we agreed in the dialogues of Part IV perhaps we could also agree that both men wished to "escape the tight conformity" of the British Psychoanalytical Society? But there is a real difference between them both in this search, it seems to me. Winnicott plunged himself into committee work and even became president of the society for a second time in 1965 – actually after Bion had been president. It was three years after his term as president that Bion left for California in January 1968, when he must have been around 73. He was a year older than Winnicott, who died before his 75th birthday, on 25 January 1971, whereas Bion was 81 when he died.

I'd love to know more about your thoughts as to why Bion made such a radical decision to leave London and move to California in 1968. It's interesting that although Winnicott did not move to America, he did wish to offer his paper "The use of an object" to the New York Institute in 1968 rather than to a Scientific Meeting of the British Psychoanalytical Society. I wonder why both men felt they would have more of an audience in America?

We started the book with some biographical notes on our protagonists, so it's fitting I think that we are now closing the book with some thoughts on their concluding aims in their psychoanalytic work.

Robert D. Hinshelwood: Yes, it is an interesting question – why did Bion abandon British psychoanalysis in 1968? And why didn't Winnicott? I know a little about Bion's decision – though not enough. Albert Mason, who was from US parents but was brought up and trained as a psychoanalyst in Britain, was instrumental in attracting Bion. He said Bion needed more money to pay his children through school in England. I am not sure whether Albert was giving the whole reason! Surely the reputation of California must have been attractive at the time in terms of its wild embrace of new ideas, Esalen, LSD, hippie freedoms; in fact, any new idea seems to have been acceptable, and Bion certainly thought he was thinking out of the box at the time. Within psychoanalysis, Brandchaft, Atwood, Stolorow, and others were turning their back (like Kohut, Fromm, and Searles) on the rigidity of instincts and drive theory. My guess is you are right that Bion was looking for a kind of freedom from institutional conformity. It was his achievement in military psychiatry (the Northfield experiment and others) in 1942–1944. Also, Bion left the Tavistock Clinic in 1948 as he thought the new NHS could be a suffocating institution (according to Dicks, 1970). I suspect, though I don't know, that there was a similar sense of potentially being stifled within the Klein group. After Klein died, Bion remained very loyal to her, unlike, I think, Winnicott and Heimann. Bion became chair of the Melanie Klein Trust and, as you mention, president of the British Psychoanalytical Society from 1962 to 1965. But it may be that after Klein died there were tensions over the need either to stick to her orthodoxy or to develop her ideas. Bion was definitely on the side of the latter.

In line with the idea of being stifled, from the mid-1960s Bion began to reject the practice of presenting or even writing up session material. Only the two people actually in the session could know what actually went on there. As I mentioned, he became less and less interested in words and semantic or symbolic meaning, and more and more interested in what minds actually do to each other. He had always been of the view that minds have a direct impact on each other, unmediated by words. He called it intuition explicitly in 1970, but it was recognisable as the influence of Jung when Bion trained at the Tavistock in the 1930s.

This is one of the major commitments he stuck to throughout his career from before he was a psychoanalyst. It is the immediate life of the session in which the analyst is a willing or unwilling partner. In my view, he found that it fits with the living dramas that Klein found in the immediate play of her children, as they were occupied with just the same pre-occupations. For Klein and Bion, Winnicott must have seemed way off track trying to excavate history, and they may have regarded it as a defensive manoeuvre that would keep the analyst out of the distracting/disturbing cut-and-thrust of the immediate drama in play. As one of Bion's early followers, Henry Ezriel, commented, "Only such forces as exist at a certain time can have effects at that time" (Ezriel, 1956, p. 35), meaning you cannot change history. This contrasts strikingly with Winnicott's surprisingly classical view, which you mention in Chapter 9, that a patient will regress to the infantile past. Actually, you also talk of Winnicott's apparently alternative commitment to interpreting the point of urgency, an idea he no doubt admired in Klein's *Psychoanalysis of Children*.

J.A.: Strange to think that Bion might have been excited by all the things that were happening in California related to the therapies that were burgeoning from psychoanalysis. It reminds me of that song that was released in 1967 by the Flower Pot Men, "Let's go to San Francisco", and how very influential it was. But things were very much changing in London too. It also had not occurred to me that Bion may have been interested in earning more money at that stage of his life and career. I suppose I had assumed that as a training analyst he would have had quite a number of analysands and supervisees. I wonder what happened to them when he decided to leave?

Winnicott had always been independently wealthy, although in the last few years of his life he was very preoccupied with money, especially after nearly dying in New York in the autumn of 1968 after having given his paper "The use of an object". I imagine the preoccupation with money (resources) was related to his fragility, as he was really quite ill up to the time he died in early 1971(Kahr, 1996, pp. 113–135). This would have contributed to Winnicott's not wishing to leave London, but my sense is it would not have occurred to him. He identified very much with being British, albeit Devonian, and although he did not have such a satisfactory time in the British Psychoanalytical Society in terms of recognition of his scientific contributions, he nevertheless was very committed to the society and its work.

Although I take your point that Bion was loyal to Melanie Klein after her death and was chair of the Klein Trust for a while as well as president of the society, perhaps his sense of incarceration was decisive for his making such a radical move from London to California. Like Winnicott, he was tired of "towing the party line". This issue of orthodoxy versus development or advance is a difficult issue in all disciplines. For psychoanalysis, the tensions continue to this day related to what constitutes psychoanalysis and what does not. How do we assess that problem when we are examining different practices, as we are between Winnicott and Bion?

As we write in 2022, the tensions going back to the Controversial Discussions still continue and can be felt, even on zoom, in almost every Scientific Meeting of the society. There is a real divide still between the three groups, even though there is a manifest protest that there are no divides. And in the Klein group, while many may celebrate and study Bion's work, the majority, I have understood, think that Bion "went wrong" when he left for California, and therefore his late work is not approved of. I think I'm right in saying this, am I not?

Bion's focus on "what minds actually do to each other", as you emphasise, unmediated by words, is not so far from Winnicott's final preoccupations. He was focusing on the "fate of aggression" in his final work and the outcome of the mother's psyche on the infant's nascent psyche. The clinical session, therefore, would inevitably bring this early history into play in the present tense of the transference on all levels of development. So this brings me to the issue about history in the session.

I don't see Winnicott's approach at "trying to excavate history", as you put it. This implies a cognitive wish on the analyst's part, which was absolutely not what Winnicott practised. I think Winnicott would have agreed with Ezriel about not being able to change history. However, his point (and also Freud's) was that analytic work can change the way the patient thinks about their history, or we could say it "manages" their history. This is fundamental to psychoanalysis, isn't it? The main aim is to strengthen the ego so that the past that rules the present can be placed in the past. How this occurs is related to what happens in the transference, which is why Winnicott did recognise the importance of "the point of urgency" – influenced not only by Klein's work but also by James Strachey, who conceptualised the "mutative interpretation". I went into this in some detail in Chapter 10 of our first book in this series (Abram and Hinshelwood, 2018, pp. 141–176).

I feel that what Bion refers to as "intuition" could be further explicated. Why was he against writing up the session material, for example? And how does "intuition" relate to the here-and-now transference? What is the difference between interpreting in the here and now and interpreting in the present tense of the transference?

R.D.H.: Bion and his wife moved to LA for multiple reasons, probably. Bion was not so British, having been in India for eight of his formative years. One suspects that he might have experienced a permanent restlessness. I was always surprised that he lived out in Croydon and travelled in to his practice and meetings and so forth. I do think he was not properly conformist. He was in trouble quite a bit in the army in WW2. He said he was the only person he knew who left at the end of the war in the same rank (major) as he entered in 1941.

I think his loyalty to Klein was at least as personal as it was professional. And I have often wondered if his dense epistemological writings about psychoanalysis as science (around 1960–1965) were an attempt to give Kleinian psychoanalysis a precise metapsychology – a part of his mourning for her (after 1960) – like Strachey did Freud's for *Works* and Jones with the biography after Freud died in 1939.

Incidentally I always wondered about Winnicott's analysis with Strachey, how long it took, and how immediately after he went for a Kleinian analysis. Do we know much about the work with Strachey? Strachey saw the analyst as an "imago", a representation in the eyes of the patient of a primary object. I think Bion's approach was different. It was really not so much about representing as actually being. Looking back at the piece of material at the end of my Chapter 10 – the patient's opening remark about not being able to do anything and about how he should have rung his mother, I can see Winnicott thinking in the "as-if" mode that mother equals the transference to Bion representing mother.

But for Bion this is absolutely not a case of the inadequate mother of decades before being brought to mind (the patient's unconscious mind) in the present. It was quite different, and was more about being and doing than representing. The not ringing up, the not doing anything today, the thinking it would "be like this" – all these comments recorded by Bion indicate something the patient was *doing* to the analyst, to Bion. One might say that hearing such comments, one's heart would sink in a sort of despair at a sense of useless non-achievement. That is to say, my words are indicating something the analyst might well have felt. We do not know exactly, but it will serve for purposes of illustration. The patient then conveys a mess, filthy smells, and so on, and he has lost his sight. One can see the temptation to describe a mother leaving the baby with a smelly nappy when she should have been clearing things up and so on. The onus is on mother, and one can see that interpreting a failing mother rather than the responsible patient might be comforting for the patient – for the analyst too, who has the chance to do something better than mother.

Bion did not take it like that; it was not a representation of bad mothering, instead it is what the patient *is*, what is left of him, filthy smells and so forth, after what the patient has done. And the session went on to demonstrate that the patient's mind fragmented things, and when Bion could show the patient how they had once linked together, then a bit of the patient's mind was restored to a more mature (reality-based) level. The patient did something to Bion – he did not represent the despair, he engaged Bion to take on the role of the despair itself. Whether I have got the exact quality of being (of the patient or of the analyst) correct is less important than trying to demonstrate the difference. For Bion, the important level of work was "beneath" the level of representation. It involved a direct impact on the analyst. To my mind, Winnicott did not clarify in his alternative description how these two levels compared, and it would have been so much easier to follow if he had actually understood Bion's level of working – and put it in relation to his own.

It is the sense of playing a role as something for the patient in his pre-occupation which is different from the interpretation of represented meanings. Psychologists at that time were talking of non-verbal communication, but Bion did not use the term, and it was not quite what he meant. He was at great pains to try to distinguish the two different forms of communication – and perhaps he never quite captured it well enough. We saw this in the quotes in Chapter 8 trying to clarify the forms of communication, and in the previous dialogue. In 1970 he clearly distinguished between the sensuous reactions of others, and the empathic knowledge of what it feels like to be anxious

He is trying to describe a direct impact on the other person (on the analyst), who can feel the feelings too. This is not just the representation of a meaning in visual, palpable signs and symbols, facial expressions, gestures. It is empathy at work.

This was the reason that Bion felt clinical reports could never do the job that was needed. Only the two in the room could have a necessary sense of the direct impact on each other's' mental experience. Of a report he gave in an earlier paper he said, ironically, in 1967:

> I cannot improve on the description I gave in that paper though it could not carry conviction to anyone who did not want to be convinced, and might well put a strain on the credulity of someone who did.
>
> (Bion, 1967, p. 196)

From the mid-1960s on, he did not publish any formal case histories and seemed uninterested in the publication of his many international clinical seminars (very many of which were recorded).

Finally on this point, one word that Bion used about this kind of direct impact was "ineffable". Some have rather inaccurately understood Bion as taking to mysticism and those supra-natural kinds of communications mystics describe. A close reading of Bion never reveals a mystical side to him. Quite the reverse: he does quote some mystics, but only to demonstrate the way his kind of intuition is prevalent in many forms of discourse, from the everyday to the aesthetic and to the supposed spiritualist. In this non-mystical form, Bion had understood this intuitive communication from way back in the early 1940s and believed it to be inherent among the ordinary human gifts.

J.A.: I was sure Bion must have lived in Hampstead if not North London somewhere, but I hadn't imagined him living in Croydon. I guessed it might have been much easier for him to leave the UK because he had lived in India for so many years in his early years, and perhaps the climate of California was also attracting him. I am not sure what you mean by him getting into trouble in the army other than having the impression that he didn't like conforming, I suppose. It's interesting that Winnicott's upbringing was in a Wesleyan Methodist religion (that is, non conformist) in Devon, and it's said that his father told him to read the Bible and then think for himself. But he embraced Darwin when he was sent to the well-known Methodist boarding school the Leys School in Cambridge when he was 14. He was twice the age Bion was when sent away to school.

Winnicott was in analysis with Strachey for ten years (1923–1933) and he was always honest about the fact that he was ill and therefore needed analysis. This was about four years after he found out that psychoanalysis existed from reading Freud's *The Interpretation of Dreams* at around the age of 23, when he had returned from being a probation medic on a destroyer in the final nine months of WW1 in 1918. He had a consultation with Ernest Jones, who referred him to James Strachey, who himself had not long returned from his analysis with Freud and was setting up in private practice. There's no doubt, as we covered in Part I of this book, that Winnicott was traumatised by WW1 and never really recovered from a sense of guilt about surviving when so many of his colleagues died. This must have also related to his early psychic development, as he would have been the first to admit.

In the obituary Winnicott wrote when James Strachey died, he said how grateful he was for that analysis and how much he had learnt (as I say in Chapter 9). Actually, it was James Strachey who recommended he go to Melanie Klein for supervision, saying he would not get from Strachey what he would get from Klein. I don't know if that inspired Winnicott to wish for a Kleinian analyst, but due to the fact that he was treating Klein's son Eric, he could not go into analysis with Klein herself (although perhaps he wanted to), and instead went into analysis with Joan Riviere for five years. I have the impression that he was not so satisfied with the latter analysis, as he felt Riviere did not accept his work on the environment, and in later years he said it took him many years to recover from her rejection of his views (Winnicott, 1989). I think this may also have contributed to his feeling so rejected by Klein on a scientific level. After the 1940s, it seems they hardly spoke, even though we know from the biographies that Klein had written a detailed letter saying how grateful she was for his treatment of her son Eric, but the letter was written in 1941 (Rodman, 2003).

But now I want to address some of the points you make about difference in technique and approach. While I've been reading what you say, I have to confess to feeling puzzled. So let me go through the sentences that puzzle me.

You say you recognise that Winnicott is thinking in the "as-if" mode when his remarks to Bion are based on his (Winnicott's) assumption that the patient's words relate to the maternal transference, that is, to a mother who failed him in his early psychic stages. I think that's right.

But then you say that for Bion it is not a question of the "as-if" mode but "rather of being and doing than representing". But from whose point of view do you mean? If you mean from the patient's point of view it is "rather of being and doing than representing", then surely you are referring to a patient who is functioning at a concrete level and demonstrating that he is not able to appreciate that his experience on the couch constitutes an "as-if" world. Is this what you mean? So the patient in question knows Bion is his analyst but he cannot really appreciate that what he feels towards him is related to his inner world. This is an example of a patient who is not able to distinguish between Me and Not-Me, and who therefore would be assessed as functioning on a borderline or psychotic level.

But surely Bion, as this psychotic patient's analyst, would know that what the patient is "doing" – (I would rather say "communicating") – *is* related to the transference, would he not? And at this level it would be described as a delusional or psychotic transference. But whether delusional or not, though, from the non-psychotic observer's point of view the transference constitutes a representation of narratives and affects. And this, from my point of view, is precisely what we see the patient struggling to communicate.

I must say I find it very difficult to see what else this can manifest other than an earnest urge to relate or communicate emanating from the very depths of this patient's unconscious. Winnicott's point in his letter to Bion, as I interpret it, is that a borderline/psychotic patient needs an analytic intervention that will show that their problems in the present tense are related to the past – and it is the past that keeps getting registered in the present because the trauma of the past cannot get to the past. The danger of the kind of abstract interventions that Bion makes is that the patient may be driven further into the psychotic world. I think this is what Winnicott means by the danger of abstract interpretations.

Nevertheless, I do understand you when you say that Bion did not see what the patient was "doing" as a representation of bad mothering but rather as what the patient feels is himself. But isn't this the psychotic functioning manifesting itself in this literal way? These layers can occur in all analyses, and I had understood this was one of the main aims of Bion's paper (that is, to show the different parts of the personality and how they function). But it is not at all clear where the non-psychotic layer of this patient was manifesting itself.

I think I also appreciate that Bion was getting to a level "beneath" that of representation and that this was the "direct impact" on the analyst. But isn't this what is understood as the unconscious impact, or non-verbal? Doesn't it also constitute the countertransference?

Being something for the patient is precisely what Winnicott describes in his work, and this particular example was with a patient to whom he said, "It is not you who is mad but me". You'll remember we discussed this in our first book and you were critical of Winnicott's position. And yet Winnicott was dealing with what the patient made him feel in the present tense of the transference, which was at the same time an actualisation or repetition of a situation that depicted a historical moment in the formation of the psyche. What else could it possibly be?

When you describe direct impact on the other person, what is the difference between this way of naming it and Freud's term "unconscious to unconscious", later referred to as countertransference? To describe it as "ineffable" is not so far from Freud's term "uncanny". "Intuition" is also a valid term, but it seems to me that Bion is sort of re-inventing the wheel by referring to a phenomenon in psychoanalysis that was already established. I wonder if this is why his late work was seen to be mystifying rather than clarifying?

R.D.H.: Yes, I can see it is difficult to explain the difference between, on the one hand, a patient working out a narrative with the analyst in such a way that they represent roles or figures that have evolved from the past, and on the other, the direct "hit" of the psychotic part of the personality. I think Bion must have constantly found that distinction difficult to get across. The difference in the countertransference is between feeling, shall we say, maternal, on one hand, and on the other finding bits and pieces of the patient's mind lodged in one's own. Could one that one were being asked not to mother the patient but rather to be a repository for refuse flung away which you, as analyst, become – the filthy things and smells?

Some people say Bion was still occupied with a WW1 battlefield in which shrapnel was flying round and could penetrate anytime as a wound into your body. Whatever the image Bion used, the analyst *is* some repudiated lost fragment of the patient's mind. It is not that the patient has represented his mother as the analyst but that some bit of the patient's mind that might have been some internalised element of his mother is now no longer internal (to the patient). The analyst has to identify the bit of the patient's mind and experience which is now lodged in them. The patient was psychotic, had "lost his mind" (in ordinary language), or he had "gone to pieces". The patient could no longer function with a coherent mind, until…

The point of Bion's vignette was that eventually a moment of functioning could be restored and he could "see" the weekend in his mind again. Of course, it is true that Bion was interpreting the psychotic part of his patient. And there was also a non-psychotic part which could understand how words represent meanings and actions and so on. And Bion, addressing the non-psychotic part that could use words, had enabled that part to gain a bit of dominance for a moment, such that the patient resumed the reality principle with Bion's supportive linking.

This is not as foreign as we might think. I can use words to communicate a meaning, an experience, a request/demand, and so forth. But words themselves can degenerate into missiles used simply to hurt rather than to carry meaning as such. If I were to shout at someone, "You fucking cunt!" (I don't often do that, I should say!), I would not be using the semantic meanings of the words "fuck" or "cunt". My aim would be to hurt, to cause a painful state of mind, a wound, to make the other person bleed. This is quite different from telling someone that I disagree with the point they have just made and that I even think they were mischievous in making it. In the latter the words retain meaning. Bion was uncompromising in saying we should always get beyond meanings and representations and discover the harm done – the full blast, as he once called it. Whether he was right or not, he thought most analysts (including Winnicott, for instance) shied away from that level of direct impact. And as you know, Bion was not the only Kleinian who thought Winnicott shied away from the destructive side, the side evident at this moment (in 2022) in Ukraine and which makes us all want to shy away from that inhumanity in ourselves.

J.A.: I don't think you're answering my questions, Bob. And it's reminding me of the IPA webinar last year (2021) when I was questioning what I felt the patient was saying and stating why I thought it would have been difficult for him to understand what Bion was saying. While I can see the "logic" behind Bion's method, I am not convinced the patient in his example shows how he has been helped when he mentions the weekend.

My impression is that this patient is very attached to Bion and has been coming for several years, and that he believes in some part of himself that Bion will help him or is helping him. But that does not mean that Bion *is* helping him. Perhaps it's true to say that we'll never know how we really help our patients, whatever technique we use.

Also – there are phases in every analysis when the analyst experiences being "used as a repository" – in fact, at some level, it occurs all the time. When you talk about the filthy things and smells flung away, surely this could be seen as relating to different developmental stages (for example, anal) in each patient depending on their history. It could also be seen as a perverse defence in action. But my point is that it conveys a communication from the patient about a layer of his psyche that is desperate to be seen and understood. And that can only occur if the analyst *receives* the bits and pieces and is really affected by them. This is all part of the psychic work the analyst has to be engaged in for every patient. But this is not an original perspective, and what I was hoping you would illuminate for me are the differences Bion was making in comparison with what is established in psychoanalysis; that is, the unconscious-to-unconscious communication and countertransference. In other words, dare I say it, I don't think Bion is so original in his way of working here.

This dialogue seems to be as difficult as the final dialogue we had in the first book, when I said the transference was illusory and you had difficulty in understanding what I meant. We were talking about different meanings of "illusion". When Freud, in 1911, wrote *The Future of an Illusion*, he was referring to "illusion" as a false perception that belonged to child development. But Winnicott enlisted the term "illusion" to denote a particular layer in the mind related to the development of perception and the capacity to discern. I realise now that this is one of the reasons why there seemed to be a misunderstanding between us during that dialogue. It's noticeable, to me, that many Kleinians do not appreciate transitional phenomena in Winnicott's work. John Steiner sees it as a psychic retreat, which is pathological, and although Ron Britton has written about imagination and reality, his work has as its foundations the Kleinian paradigm, which does not account, I think, for the layer of the transference that constitutes illusion – not delusion or disillusion – but rather illusion emanating from the deepest layers of the psyche that relates to the history of the psyche even though the latter may not be interpreted in a cognitive way. De facto, the psyche has a history that reverberates constantly, and the analysing situation provokes specific underlying historical events and traumas. The problem, for me, with the here-and-now interpreting is that it seems to delete history – which in turn constitutes deleting the reality principle, because there is a propensity to negate development and history. In and of itself this is maddening.

Your example of shouting abuse at someone and using words to hurt or cause pain does not take account of anxiety in the patient's communication. I think when this happens in analysis it signifies that the transference has evolved to such a point of intensity that the patient may not be able to retain a sense of reality and time is distorted. It means something different for each patient and is not necessarily aimed at hurting or maiming. It could be a sign of identification with the aggressor. I can think of one patient who terrified me with this kind of abuse, and it took me some time to realise that he was his father shouting at me, who at that moment was standing in for himself or another. The main aim in the analysis, albeit unconscious I believe, was to get me to feel something that he had felt when witnessing his father shout at him and/or others. This is a very common example, and I think it would be called projective identification in Kleinian terminology, wouldn't it?

Do you have a reference for the claim that Bion thought Winnicott "shied away" from a direct level of impact? This seems to me to refer to a publication in which Winnicott was accused of not being able to analyse Masud Khan's aggression. This was, in my view, "wild analysis". And it was also based on Khan's fabrications about the length of time he was in analysis with Winnicott. This wild analysis, based on fabrications, has been addressed by research in the Winnicott archives and was published in the bulletin of the society in 2018 (Abram, Joyce, and Thompson, 2018; 2022). What the article highlights is the way in which this kind of myth can be exploited to discredit Winnicott – something that has been going on for many years and which, I thought, we were trying to avoid in our series.

Clinical psychoanalysis has aimed to address personal aggression, hate, sadism, and death wishes since Freud started. Klein and her followers do not have the monopoly on understanding the very dangerous aspects in all personalities. In fact, it is psychoanalysis from every clinical paradigm, in my view, that helps us understand the roots of war. As analysts, we are trying to confront differences and compare and contrast the different ways of working. While I understand Winnicott's letter to Bion about that piece of clinical work, as I've tried to explain, I accept that at the same time I have no way of knowing which technique is the most helpful. But I do know that when I read Bion's account I feel concerned for the patient because I think, rather I felt, that he did not know what was going on and was feeling mad – I would venture to say – in a mad environment (constituted, that is, by Bion's way of talking to him).

R.D.H.: Yes, it may be that I did not answer your questions well, but I did say that I think Bion himself had difficulty in getting across the distinction between communication and the deeper level he was trying to describe. Some ten years after that particular case material, Bion did, as I mentioned, believe that his presentations would stretch anyone's credulity. And he largely gave up case presentation. Only those present could feel the blast of the patient's projections, and perhaps only those present could comment on the blasting of the analyst's – and the patient's – mind.

I do understand that Winnicott was committed to the view that someone else in the environment was responsible for the condition of the patient's mind and troubles. Of course, the environment is extremely important. As Ernest Jones (1935) once said, no one will deny the importance of the environment and nurture, but what psychoanalysis has to offer is an understanding of the internal meanings and inherent struggles of the patient as an added factor; a significant added factor because it is unconscious.

And even if the patient is responsible to a significant degree for his own troubles, his carers should be responsible for recognising the patient's own internal responsibility as a baby, and I suppose that includes his present-day analyst.

The answer I was trying to get across to you and the readers involves Bion's differentiation between communication (including unconscious-to-unconscious communication) and something different. The object of the difference is what Bion was trying to elaborate from Klein's original description of the ego-weakness that comes from a self-destructive splitting. The work Kleinians did with psychotic states was focused on that damage to the ego, which needs some reconstitution before it can represent things, before it can communicate, and before it can tackle conflicts such as the oedipal ones or earlier forms, including anal ones, as you suggest. Klein's initial description, back in the 1930s, was of this early destructiveness that eventually resolved, in her later conceptualisation, into splitting. The ensuing split-off bits were then dealt with by evacuation, simple expulsion; the getting rid of what felt then like mental refuse. A term that was in vogue at one time was "lavatory mother".

Bion conceived, however, a different form from evacuative-projective identification. It has come to be called container-contained. He was not the only analyst to consider this a sort of projective communication. It is different from an evacuation – a getting rid of fragments of the mind just to get rid of them, anywhere, without thought of communication. What the analyst can hope to do, when he is on form, is to lever those evacuated pieces into some restored representation that can have a communicative property. You said that there was no evidence in the material that Bion did anything other than miss the point. But there is evidence. He did his best to collect fragments into some connection again. And it had a confirming result: the patient could recognise a moment of reality. It is this response that Bion regarded as confirmation. Of course, Winnicott could not get a confirmation because he did not give his interpretation to the patient. It does seem a little presumptuous to quarrel with Bion's interpretation when there was empirical confirmation. Of course, one could argue that Bion's understanding of the response to his interpretation is not valid, but that was not what Winnicott took up. For instance, in your own example, where you represented the patient's shouting father, what was your observed confirmation that you were correct?

Freud (1911) identified the capacity to handle reality as the significant defect in psychotic states. You know his view that in human development a capacity to inhibit motor action (which dominates animal mentation) opens a space for thinking as an "experimental form of action", as he put it. This capacity for the reality principle is a core element of the ego – even in his later structural model in 1923 – and Bion was very influenced by that 1911 paper on the reality principle.

I don't know of any reference Bion made to Winnicott's view on destructiveness; in fact, he more or less completely ignored Winnicott – rather uncivil, in my view. Actually, I did not have in mind the Masud Khan problem for Winnicott. I had in mind you own view that Winnicott could not contemplate the death instinct in terms of inner object relations. For Winnicott, destructiveness was always, and only, due to the failing environment and never a feature of the personality from the beginning, as Klein (and thus Bion) assumed. The inherent capacity to hate, comparable to the inherent capacity to love, was inconceivable for Winnicott – I believe I took this from you. I think Klein and Winnicott diverged in their fundamental assumptions. Winnicott thought there was only love until the infant comes up against an intractable other, and for Klein, the capacity to hate a difficult other is as inherent as loving a loving other. Unless one recognises the differing unspoken assumptions, it is easy to talk past each other rather than engage; as Bion once remarked: "Controversy is the growing point from which development springs, but it must be a genuine confrontation and not an impotent beating of the air by opponents whose differences of view never meet" (Bion, 1970, p. 55). It would not surprise me if Bion had Winnicott in mind, given the discourtesies between them. Their differences start with Bion's view that back in infancy, hate is an inherent state parallel to love, with which Winnicott disagreed. On that basis, diverging from Klein, and indeed from the late Freud, Winnicott needed to establish other underlying assumptions – the infant's initial non-experience of another, the singular responsibility of the environment for personality distortions, and the psychotic existential problems. This may be at the root of Winnicott's idiosyncratic use of the term "the illusion of omnipotence".

Maybe, Jan, this clarifies some things, even if only differences and their prickly relations!

J.A.: There's no doubt, Bob, that the clinical experience of a psychoanalytic treatment is difficult to convey to people who have never undergone psychoanalysis. The psychoanalytic literature from Freud's case studies onwards aims to illustrate evidence that the psychoanalytic method works for emotional disorders, and to a large extent it has been successful if we look at the international proliferation of psychoanalysis for the past hundred years.

It's interesting that Bion decided that his clinical examples would "stretch anyone's credulity". I find myself questioning the perspective that only those present could know about the "blasting of the analyst's mind". This does not seem to me to take account of the way in which the unconscious communicates from one person to another – especially if the other is a seasoned analyst. I am thinking of two specific situations – 1) one to one supervision, and 2) inter-analytic clinical group work.

When supervising, we listen to the communication from the analyst who discusses the case, who often brings a verbatim session. We pick up on the meaning of the transmissions from analysand to analyst and we comment. The supervisee is more often than not surprised and relieved that the supervisor is able to articulate something that has been difficult to reveal. The supervisory relationship evolves, and the supervisor, like a co-parent, attunes themselves to the clinical issues that arise during the course of the treatment. I know that what I'm writing about is nothing new for you, Bob, but I wanted to set out something to highlight the essential need to share clinical work with others. It's not just the supervisory relationship, of course. I have ongoing continual professional development (CPD) meetings, and there is always something that I learn about myself and my patients. This is the very reason CPD is so essential in our work.

Let me also briefly mention what I mean by inter-analytic clinical group work. I was involved in an European Psychoanalytical Federation research group for many years in which an analyst brings two to three consecutive sessions with no history of the patient or history of the course of the analysis. The group listens to the session and formulates the history of the patient and the history of the analysis by simply saying aloud feelings and thoughts evoked by the material in the group work. These meetings over the course of a day and a half clearly show how different aspects of the analytic pair can be communicated to each and every member of the group. We came to name this "diffraction", which is a particular type of transference. In a paper (Abram, 2014) in which I detail this experience, I suggested the notion of an inter-analytic mirror that evolves out of this kind of research group. Because of your longstanding involvement in groups, a lot of what I'm saying will resonate for you, along with Bion's work on groups too, of course. This is why I find it puzzling that he eschewed the need to communicate clinical work in his later years.

Winnicott did believe categorically that the mother's mind had a crucial and long-lasting impact on the nascent psyche, but he also believed that the baby brought something innate into the relationship; that is, inherited tendencies. It's always nature and nurture for Winnicott, and I think Bion also agreed with this after he had formulated the container-contained theory. And I do think I appreciate the difference between a kind of pure discharge "evacuation" and a more thought-out communication from the patient in the consulting room. Nevertheless, when being used as a lavatory mother, I feel the analyst has to work on the underlying communication, which inevitably, in my view, is historical.

You asked me how did I know that the patient was treating me in the transference in the way his father had treated him in the past? It's beyond the scope of this dialogue to go into much detail except to say that it took me many years of psychic work in that analytic treatment to not only think but feel that my observation, based on the terrifying feelings I had to endure, convinced me not that I was right specifically but that it made sense. But it was also true that at the point I could start to feel less terrified in the sessions, I was able to respond differently. This made all the difference to the patient, and I came to think of Strachey's mutative interpretation and how it changes something very fundamental for the patient. Instead of the analyst being the patient's archaic object, the mutative interpretation means the patient is able to perceive the analyst as someone different – in other words, as the helpful other. The analysis changed from that moment onward, which confirmed to me that some of my observations were plausible (Abram, 2022, pp. 59–76). I am guessing we are not a million miles apart about this.

Winnicott did not see the death instinct as a useful concept. This is addressed in our first book in Chapters 7 and 8 (Abram and Hinshelwood, 2018). But it's not that Winnicott was shying away from the emotions of death wishes, murderousness, hate, sadism, and so on. It's more that he saw those affects as developmental achievements in the baby rather than as affects they could possibly feel in their earliest moments of being born. In other words, he felt that Klein imbued the infant with sophisticated affects that had not yet evolved in the psyche. This is the main difference in Winnicott and Bion's basic assumptions. The infant does have an initial experience right from the start, and the environment is not totally responsible for the infant's evolving pathology – there is always an admixture of inherited tendencies and the mother's psyche – but the latter certainly has a powerful impact on inherited tendencies. I think the term "illusion of omnipotence" is an apt way of depicting how the mother's adaptation to the newborn infant's needs makes the baby feel like God. But she then has to help the baby to realise they *are not* God – little by little. This is the immense power she has.

It is a mystery to me why Bion was rather uncivil to Winnicott on a scientific level. This kind of negation of a colleague's co-current work is not acceptable nowadays, although, regardless, it unfortunately still occurs.

Perhaps we now have to leave this dialogue and let the reader work out how they understand the differences and how they wish to think about their specific uses of the objects we have been setting out in our second book of the series. What do you think, Bob?

GLOSSARY

This glossary is based on the glossary in the first book of the series – *The Clinical Paradigms of Melanie Klein and Donald Winnicott: Comparisons and Dialogues*. The aim is to define some of the specific terms that are used throughout the book by both Robert D. Hinshelwood and Jan Abram. For more in-depth definitions of Kleinian and Winnicottian terms the reader is advised to turn to the two main textbooks by the present authors – Hinshelwood's *A Dictionary of Kleinian Thought* (1989) and Abram's 2nd edition of *The Language of Winnicott* (2007).

Aggression

JAN ABRAM: Winnicott conceptualises aggression at the start of life as synonymous with activity and motility. He refers to "primary aggression" and states that instinctual aggressiveness is originally part of appetite. So this is a concept of benign aggression, which is the engine of the life instinct. Aggression changes in quality as the infant develops and the change will absolutely depend on the kind of environment in which the infant finds themself. With good-enough mothering, aggression becomes integrated into the personality and sense of self. But if the environment fails, aggression will manifest itself in a destructive and/or antisocial way. Winnicott's concept of aggression evolved and in his late work it is pivotal to all the most celebrated of his concepts – the antisocial tendency, creativity, the good-enough mother, transitional phenomena, true and false self, and finally, the use of an object (Abram, 2007, pp. 15–40; Abram, 2013, ch. 14; Abram, 2022).

ROBERT D. HINSHELWOOD: Bion followed Klein in seeing aggression as the origin of anxiety from the beginning. The initial ego is primed to recognise others beyond its boundary, and the confusion or conflict of love and hate towards them creates primary anxiety. Initially, this arises from the need for bodily satisfaction but invades the mental domain as personal experiences of others develop, and Bion endorsed Klein's pointed descriptions of envy. Bion saw this primary anxiety as one that requires the other person/carer to process it before the subject can do it for themselves (see "container-contained"). The growth of a mind comes from its taking on the ability to process unknown or painful experiences (see "alpha-function"). Bion's interest was less in the nature of these experiences that need processing and more in that alpha-function process together with the kind of intuitive/evoking process necessary for achieving alpha-function. He also focused extensively and deeply on the obstructions to and destruction of alpha-function, and therefore on the inhibition of growth.

Alpha-element

Alpha-elements are meaningful entities that are produced by alpha-function and the basic elements used by the mind and its functioning (see "alpha-function" and "container-contained").

Alpha-function

Bion's theory of making meanings involves several functions. The first is a perception or a sensation he called a beta-element. Then, secondly, this is elaborated in the mind in relation to previous similar experiences or a newly evolved meaning; this he called alpha-function. The result, the third step, is that the product of alpha-function is an alpha-element, which is usable in dreams, thoughts and memories. Where alpha-function fails, the original beta-element remains meaningless and unusable and often feels persecuting (eliciting a nameless dread) (see "container-contained" and "internal object").

Anxiety (psychic pain)

J.A.: For Winnicott, there were two fundamental qualities to the subjective experience of anxiety, and both were caused by the psychic (environment). If the (psychic) environment was deficient at the earliest stages of life, then primitive and unthinkable anxieties occurred. The deficient early environment therefore led to psychotic defences. Due to a good-enough environment, the second quality of anxiety was oedipal – that is, castration anxiety.

R.D.H.: Bion adopted Klein's descriptions of the two basic forms of anxiety: the fear for one's survival (paranoid-schizoid position), and the fear of harming or destroying loved and needed others (depressive position). But Bion focused almost exclusively on the first of these, the disintegration of the self/ego.

Clinical paradigm

J.A.: The term "paradigm" follows the groundbreaking work of Thomas Kuhn, who published *The Strucure of Scientific Revolutions* in 1962. Kuhn's theory of scientific revolutions has been used by Zeljko Loparic, a Brazilian philosopher, to understand the "paradigm change" from Freud to Winnicott (Abram, 2013).

We have added the term "clinical" for the title of this book to emphasise the crucial nature of clinical practice that, for both Klein and Winnicott, was the sine qua non of the formulation of psychoanalytic theories and technique. Thus a clinical paradigm refers to a set of guiding principles that are founded on clinical practice.

Concern

J.A.: Winnicott largely agreed with Melanie Klein's conceptualisation of the depressive position and refers to this term in many of his writings up to 1960. However, in his late work, after 1960, he revised Klein's theory by focusing on how the infant comes to acquire a "capacity" for concern. Winnicott's emphasis on the development of the capacity for concern relates to the coming together of the environment and object mother. This description differs from Klein's stress, followed by Bion, on the "good" and the "bad" division in the mind of the paranoid-schizoid position.

R.D.H.: Bion focused mostly on Klein's paranoid-schizoid position, and thus rarely paid attention to reparation and depressive anxiety, though he acknowledged how concern evolved out of the paranoid-schizoid division of love.

Container-contained

R.D.H.: This term was developed by Wilfred Bion from about 1959; the term was taken from Jung. However, the concept is so closely connected to Klein's major discovery of projective identification that containing cannot be separated today from Kleinian psychoanalysis.

The idea is that psychological development proceeds from the very earliest days through a process by which mother/carer will internalise the baby's mental states – when the baby cries, for instance, and the mother becomes alarmed – and proceed to give those a meaning. She then conveys the meaning to the baby through appropriate action – feeding if the baby is crying with hunger. The baby learns by this process what meaning its sensations have.

There are many similarities between Bion's concept of container-contained and Winnicott's concept of holding (see "holding"). The distinctions and similarities were presented in Part III.

Countertransference

J.A.: Winnicott was one of the first analysts to develop the concept of countertransference when he published "Hate in the countertransference" in 1947. In this paper he differentiated between three types of countertransference, including one that was psychopathological and meant the analyst required more analysis. His clinical example in the paper highlights the way in which he used his countertransference in clinical work. The main argument was that the affect "hate" has to be acknowledged by the analyst when working with the psychotic patient, otherwise the hate engendered will lead to serious acting out on the part of the clinician (analyst and/or psychiatrist). Lobotomy and leucotomy were practices Winnicott saw as "acting out".

R.D.H.: Initially (always) a phenomenon of disputed worth. Originally, Freud and his colleagues viewed the analyst's emotional responses to his patients with deep suspicion, as Jung, Ferenczi, and other colleagues were drawn into quite suspect behaviour. A number of analysts in the 1930s, including Marjorie Brierley and John Rickman, focused on the analyst's emotional reactions and their behaviour, which set the scene for a revision during the 1940s. Rickman influenced Bion strongly in the use Bion made of his own countertransference experience of being pushed into a role in his work with groups from 1943 onwards. From 1946, Bion was supervised by Paula Heimann during his psychoanalytic training.

Increasingly, as Bion developed his understanding of intuition as the prime mode of communication that the analyst should attend to, the introspection that is synonymous with working with the countertransference became more important. Countertransference is the intuitive receptiveness involved in the container-contained relationship in a session which is the important function for the psychoanalyst.

Death instinct

J.A.: Winnicott rejected both the Freudian and the Kleinian concepts of the death instinct. It was perhaps the one main disagreement he had with Sigmund Freud, which he referred to in his very late work (Winnicott, 1969a). In his last writings, Winnicott followed the Greek philosopher Empedocles, who had proposed a love/strife force that, like fire, could be constructive or destructive (Winnicott, 1969). Abram has proposed that Winnicott's work on the use of an object in his final three years elaborated an alternative theory to the symbolic meaning of the death instinct (Abram, 2013, ch. 14).

R.D.H.: Although Klein used the term "death instinct", Bion clarified that for him it meant the paranoid-schizoid anxiety of fearing for one's survival and arose from dependence on a frustrating object needed for the supply of food and love, or from the schizoid defences which tend to dismantle the self (see "paranoid-schizoid position"). These are innate reactions endowed from the beginning, just as with Freud's description of libido deriving from stimulation of the erogenous zones.

Bion also followed Klein in the view that all innate endowments and their development are experienced as unconscious phantasy (in the very young they are perhaps consciously experienced). Whatever the fear of fragmentation and for survival actually feels like for the infant, it can be subsumed under the adult conception of death.

Environment

J.A.: Up until 1923, Freud's work focused on the topographical model of the mind, which did not take account of the subject's environment. Rather it was psychosexuality in relation to the instincts that shaped the personality. In 1923, Freud introduced the "structural model" when he wrote *The Ego and the Id* and revised his perspective on the environment, referring to the ego having three masters: the id, the superego, and the external world (that is, the parents). In the early 1940s, Winnicott came to see that "there was no such thing as a baby" but only a baby in relation to a crucial m/other. This observation led Winnicott to formulate a theory of the environment-individual setup suggested as his first major theoretical achievement (Abram, 2008).

R.D.H.: Klein is much castigated for neglecting the effect of the social environment, but Bion is often held to correct this apparent omission with his model of container-contained (see "container-contained").

Envy

J.A.: Winnicott concurred with Klein that unacknowledged envy caused deep problems that led to psychopathology. Envy that could be acknowledged, like hate and sadism, were affects that evolved in the individual in relation to the environment. Therefore, Winnicott would say that these affects are developmental achievements and in health would be integrated into the personality. But for the ill individual envy may be a driving force and a powerful aspect of severe disturbance.

R.D.H.: Bion's paper (published in 1959) introducing the formal model of container-contained was presented to the British Psychoanalytical Society in 1957, the year that Klein published her book on envy, which dismayed so many colleague analysts. Half of that paper gives very short vignettes of destructive attitudes to dependent relations on loved others (see "psychotic anxiety"). The second half of the paper then discusses Klein's concept of destructive envy and gives a fragment of clinical evidence for the containing relationship, which Bion then develops as a model (see "container-contained"). The destructiveness is provoked by the dependence on the capacity and strength of the object to contain. It demonstrates the humiliating weakness and dependency of an infant often absorbed in its own omnipotence. That challenge leads to the hatred of envy. Much is lost in futile debates about the innateness of envy as if it occurs without stimulation (in contrast to other innate endowments) (see "death instinct").

External object

J.A.: Winnicott's work from 1945 onwards develops the notion of the environment-individual setup. The individual self, therefore, is inscribed with the earliest environment. The parent-infant relationship plays a crucial role in shaping the internal world of each individual. In this sense, the external object plays a part in the development of the sense of self, but Winnicott's stress is on what the infant and growing child "makes" of their environment. The external object is "created" by each individual. The environment-individual setup will be played out at unconscious levels in the analytic setting and constitutes the transference-countertransference matrix.

R.D.H.: Bion was not a child analyst and accepted Klein's assumption of the innateness of the ego-boundary. Therefore, external objects (real or imagined) are present from the beginning. In this most primitive of stages, the outside world is experienced as an external object given a characterisation by the state the baby feels itself to be in. If comfortable, the external object is felt to be "good"; if uncomfortable, it is felt to be "bad". Thus bodily states determine how the external object is seen, until distance perception can begin to give a truer picture, which being painful brings in the anxiety and dynamics of the depressive position, whereby another person can be felt conflictually as having *both* good and bad parts (see "anxiety (psychic pain)", "concern").

Holding

J.A.: All the details of maternal care just before birth and immediately afterwards go towards making up the holding environment. This includes the mother's primary maternal preoccupation, which is at the heart of the holding environment and enables the mother to provide the infant with the necessary ego-support at the beginning of life. Physical holding is meaningless without an emotionality of sensitivity and care that will be internalised bodily and emotionally by the infant. Holding includes the mother's mirror role in early development, which means she is able to mirror the infant's affects due to her deep identification with the infant's predicament of absolute dependence. Holding is often associated with containing but should not be confused with Bion's container-contained concept. Both concepts have similarities but emanate from different theoretical paradigms – the container-contained is based on the Kleinian paradigm, in contrast to holding, which is a concept founded on Winnicott's paradigm (see Part III).

Illusion (of omnipotence)

J.A.: The roots of imagination are initiated as a result of the baby feeling that he gets what he needs. The mother's capacity to tune into his early needs, which are both physical and emotional, helps the baby feel he has created the world. The capacity to play is predicated on the success of the baby feeling as if he were God.

R.D.H.: The nature of illusion is at the root of imagination, symbolisation, and culture. Illusion is the capacity to present one "thing" as if it were another. When this capacity is used for symbolisation, the symbol represents another as if it were the very thing it represents, without one's losing the knowledge that the representation is actually different from thing it represents. We use words as if they were what the words mean, while also knowing that words and what they mean are actually different (see "symbolisation").

Inscription

J.A.: This is a term taken from French psychoanalysis. Following Roussillon, Abram states that through the early parent-infant relationship the infant's growing sense of self is inscribed by the parental psychic responses to every aspect of dependency and development (see Chapter 2). Thus, every single person has aspects of the early environment inscribed in their sense of self which could be said to be the psychic equivalent of genetic continuity.

Internal object

J.A.: While Winnicott used the notion of the internal object, he did not agree that it was a given from the beginning of life. Rather, he saw that after a certain amount of "needs-being-adapted-to", the infant internalises the effects of the parent-infant relationship; that is, an internal object is formed through a process of internalisation rather than being an innate internal object.

Winnicott proposed the notion of a subjective object that was a product of the earliest parent-infant relationship when the mother was in a state of primary maternal preoccupation during the phase of absolute dependence. Abram has proposed that through the mother's psychic *survival-of-the-object* there evolves an intrapsychic subjective surviving object. The corollary is that through the mother's psychic non *survival-of-the-object* an intrapsychic non surviving-object evolves (see Abram, 2022, chs. 2–3).

R.D.H.: As a Kleinian, Bion accepted the primary division of an internal world from an external one. This was marked too by Karl Abraham, who placed emphasis on the mechanisms of introjection and projection. These mechanisms indicate the imagined phantasy that mental contents can be transported from inside to outside and vice versa. Working with psychotic states in the 1950s, Bion was emphatic about the importance of the role of these two mechanisms. He understood that in such states mental contents are experienced as material lumps and the phantasies of introjection and projection are modelled for the infant (and the deeper layers of the unconscious) on feeding and defecating. However, he also noted that the processes of evacuation and internalisation could occur for the psychotic mind through the various portals of the distance receptors. Thus, visual hallucinations were phantasies of ejection through the eyes, and auditory hallucinations via the ears. Those organs, in the process of vision and hearing, were felt to receive into the ego solid entities. Such concretely perceived mental entities Bion labelled beta-elements (see "alpha-function").

However, in a more normal state of mind, we "see" a world of objects displaced in relation to each other in a world around us, and we actually know that they are representations in our mind which have meanings resulting from alpha-functions that create mental experiences (see "alpha-function", "alpha-elements"). At an unconscious level there is still a sense of these objects as concrete "parts" of our bodies. They give rise to actual bodily sensations (good or bad) according to the unconscious belief in the intentions of the object. The capacity to understand these perceptions and sensations as representative of what we have seen or heard is lost in psychotic states. Internal objects, when understood as representations, are a resource for recognising meaningful things in the real world. Their regression to concrete physical entities is one fundamental dynamic of psychotic states (see "paranoid-schizoid position").

Interpretation

J.A.: While Winnicott saw interpretation as one of the principle elements of analytic practice, he lay stress on the analyst's taking account of the patient's ability to receive the interpretation and their capacity to play (that is, free associate). If the patient cannot play, then the analyst has to facilitate understanding through interpretative comments. In his late work, Winnicott privileged the holding environment in any given analysis, which should provide the incremental steps towards the analyst's mutative interpretation. While this followed Strachey's argument concerning the therapeutic action of analysis, Winnicott emphasised the analyst's ability to facilitate the patient's discovery of self through the transitional space and transferential elements at the heart of analytic practice.

R.D.H.: Conscious insight into unconscious conflicts and anxieties has been, from Freud's earliest work, the core tool of psychoanalysis and the element that distinguishes it from suggestive and other therapies. Bion, however, took this understanding a step further. The understanding that needs to be acquired via interpretation is an increase in the capacity to process our experiences (see "alpha-function") and achievement Bion called growth. Understanding of the nature of interpretation is therefore enhanced by the model of the container-contained, whereby the analyst lends their own capacity to process experiences and thus enhances the patient's capacity to contain their experiences (see "container-contained"). Bion described this as a particular relational link between two minds, which he initially labelled "K", though later he preferred the notation "O", indicating it is more than intellectual knowing and is a form of becoming (or being) each other's experiences and functions. This entails having the feelings appropriate to the other while recognising they belong to the other and are not one's own feelings (see "countertransference").

Object use

See "survival-of-the-object".

Omnipotence

J.A.: Winnicott used the term "omnipotence" to refer to the infant's feeling that they are God when their needs are met (see "illusion (of omnipotence)". This follows the notion put forwards by Freud "His majesty the baby". But this should be distinguished from the patient's omnipotent manic defence, which Winnicott would say emanates from a deficiency of early illusion (of omnipotence). The latter experience is essential for the infant to feel he has created the object.

Paranoid-schizoid position

J.A.: Winnicott thought that Klein's paranoid-schizoid position was a vivid description of a psychotic state of mind that was often mobilised in adult patients due to the analytic setting. However, he disagreed that this description could be transposed to the state of mind of the newborn infant, which led to his phrase "Early is not deep". The newborn infant had not accumulated enough experience of the parent-infant relationship to be capable of this state of mind. Moreover, the infant who was fortunate enough to have a good-enough mother/environment would benefit from a very different environment from that depicted by the paranoid-schizoid position. For Winnicott, the paranoid-schizoid position was a good description of an infant who had suffered a significant deficiency in their early environment.

R.D.H.: Bion paid relatively little attention to the depressive position (in marked contrast to Winnicott) and focused on the paranoid-schizoid position, the anxiety about surviving, and the process of the splitting of the self and its associated mechanisms. Klein's late emphasis on splitting comes after a long discussion by Edward Glover, Melitta Schmideberg (Klein's daughter), and Marjorie Brierley about disintegration of the self, following Freud's description of the splitting of the ego in his paper on "Fetishism" in 1927.

Klein emphasised the self-splitting implicit in Freud's paper. It is an act of the ego itself to split off a function that is causing pain and anxiety. Such splitting is quite different from a mental conflict. The latter may be dealt with by repressing one side of the conflict but results in a substitute formation for the repressed element, which constitutes a neurotic dynamic. In contrast, the split-off part of the ego disappears altogether, leaving a blankness of mind. That lost part of the ego is then located elsewhere and outside the ego-boundary; frequently it is believed to exist within someone else (see "projective identification").

Splitting processes also attack objects, usually to identify them as all-good (idealised) or else as evil and demonic. And similarly, processes of projection and introjection locate the object (usually a bad one) outside the self. These various processes constitute the schizoid mechanisms felt unconsciously as very concrete phantasies. At first, a mixed object, with good and bad aspects, is seen as two objects, one good and one bad. This leads to intense experiences of rather pure feelings. In particular, the bad object with intentions to harm or kill the self arouses great terror, and children of some years may show this in what is called *pavor nocturnus*, or night terrors. Similarly, the good object, which intends the infant to survive and flourish, is experienced with great bliss. As the child matures, they will see their own reactions at war with each other, the solution being that splitting of the self.

Guilt is a good example which demonstrates another important feature of the paranoid-schizoid position. A person avoids a feeling of being guilty for something by, in effect, splitting off their conscience. They may then attribute the guilt to someone else (a projective defence), and that other person can make a "counter-accusation" attributing guilt back to the subject who had projected it (see "projective identification").

Primary maternal preoccupation

J.A.: This is a term that Winnicott used to describe the state of mind the mother normally goes into just before giving birth and for the early weeks of her infant's life. The infant's healthy development is contingent on the mother's ability to go into this state of mind in which she is completely identified with the infant's predicament of dependence.

Projective identification

A basic process in the mind is the process of the splitting of the ego (see "paranoid-schizoid position"), in which a function of the ego is separated and stops functioning. This function may then be relocated in someone else – a process called projective identification. For instance, a baby may scream because it has a feeling in its tummy, and its mother not only hears the scream, she also feels the alarm that the baby feels. Or an adolescent, when asked by a parent if he has done his homework, just shrugs his shoulders, leaving the parent to worry about getting the homework done. Or someone who bumps their car into someone else's shouts accusations to ensure that the other driver embodies all the guilt for the bum.

Psyche-in-dwelling-in-the-soma

J.A.: This describes the successful outcome of the process Winnicott called "personalisation", which comes about as a result of the mother's handling during the phase of absolute dependence. Psyche connotes the "imaginative elaboration of somatic parts, feelings and functions" and is often synonymous with "fantasy", "inner reality" and "self". Psychosomatic illness is a symptom of something having gone wrong in the individual's early emotional development usually due to a deficiency in the environment (Winnicott, 1958, pp. 243–254).

Psychic creativity

J.A.: Winnicott refers to a creative drive, which Abram interprets as an extension of Freud's notion of the life instinct. It is the mother's ability to adapt to her infant's needs that facilitates the baby's feeling that they have created the object. This is the place from which the sense of self grows. Primary psychic creativity is associated with the female element in Winnicott's late work and is the basis for "creative living" and "feeling real".

Psychic pain (anxiety)

R.D.H.: James Strachey's seminal paper on interpretation in 1934, "The nature of the therapeutic action of psychoanalysis", refers to the focus of the interpretation as "the point of urgency" in the material. It directs attention to the affective moments of the session at least as much as to the thematic content of the associations. It seems likely that this was influenced by Klein at the time, who was interested in the point of anxiety.

Psychic transitionality

Abram's term used to denote the emotional journey related to "creating the object" and illusion. It refers to an evolving capacity to play and evolve in the analysing situation.

Psychotic anxiety

R.D.H.: The Kleinian interest is mainly in a layer of the unconscious that underlies the neurotic unconscious that Freud discovered and consistently elaborated. Klein had been tempted to term it the "psychotic layer", as opposed to Freud's "neurotic layer". Bion, with colleagues, worked with actual psychotic states, and showed that even in normal development the fear of disintegration (see "death instinct") could lead to further splitting and other schizoid defences. However, Bion particularly showed the difference between the splitting and projective identification that occurs in more stable personalities and an actual psychotic state encountered in psychiatry. In the psychotic state, split-off parts are desperately evacuated together with beta-elements, felt as a concrete expulsion of entities that are hardly mental, with the consequent impossible task of retrieving those bits and pieces to restore the mind. While in the normal, deeper unconscious beneath the neurotic level the evacuation is not of this excessive kind felt in physical terms, the aim is specifically at another mind capable (hopefully) of containing what the subject cannot (see "container-contained" and "projective identification").

J.A.: In Winnicott's frame of reference, psychotic anxieties relate to the deficiency in holding at the earliest stages of life. The causes of psychotic anxieties are directly associated with the psychic environmental deficiencies which cause early psychic trauma. Winnicott, in the 1940s, developed a theory of birth trauma (Winnicott, 1949; compare Abram, 2021).

Reality principle

R.D.H.: It is characteristic of psychiatric patients in psychotic states that they lose touch with their external reality – and by splitting themselves they lose touch with their internal reality. Bion turned to Freud's (1911) paper on the reality principle and the six or seven ego-functions that come into play to form that principle. This was important for Bion, as he could understand the loss of reality in terms of the splitting off of one or more of these functions. Bion's work with psychotic states involved describing to the patient the fate of these split-off functions as if they were bits of the physical body.

J.A.: Winnicott followed Freud in his theory of the reality principle, but his advance on Freud's paper on the two principles of mental life was to introduce the concept of transitional phenomena – a third principle of the mind that André Green referred to as "tertiary processes".

Response to interpretation

J.A.: Analysis with James Strachey (the author of "The nature of the therapeutic action of psychoanalysis") for ten years made a significant contribution to the way in which Winnicott worked with interpretation and his ability to listen to the patient's response. In his late work he advocated waiting for the patient before or after an interpretation so as not to pre-empt the patient's discovery of self (Winnicott, 1969).

R.D.H.: The repeated attacks that Klein and her followers faced from 1927 until her death in 1960 and after led these analysts to attempt to show how analytic work in the form of classical interpretation really changes something, bringing the session more to life. The success of an interpretation is not simply a facile "yes" in agreement but an authentic lively response. It is something that tallies with the unconscious of the patient (see "interpretation"). Such an unconscious change in the transference, felt in the countertransference, can be recognised in various ways. For Bion it took the form of an enhancement of alpha-function by which the mental capacities and functions develop or are returned from projective destinations. This especially took the form of a greater intuitive sense of connection with the patient and an enhanced ability for the patient to "be" his own understanding of his experiences.

Schizoid mechanisms/splitting

R.D.H.: Klein's seminal paper in 1946, "Notes on some schizoid mechanisms" has inspired generations of Kleinian analysts ever since. The splitting of the self was understood to be the underlying problem of psychotic states, but it has its more benign variants in all of us living ordinary lives in ordinary relationships. Splitting is directed at objects which have mixed characteristics, some good, some bad. These are typically separated into two objects, one seen as good, the other as bad. This resolves a conflict whereby one has to feel good feelings towards the good characteristics and at the same time bad feelings towards the bad characteristics of the same object. Thus, conflict can be avoided by splitting the object in this way.

Further, the ego can split itself, as Freud had originally described in 1927. Klein held a view that such self-disintegration is likely to be prominent in psychotic states. And this was confirmed by young colleagues who took on schizophrenic patients for psychoanalysis, such as Herbert Rosenfeld, who began analysis with "Mildred" in his training in 1943. Splitting of the self into non-communicating parts is assisted and supported by further mechanisms, including projective identification (see "projective identification", "paranoid-schizoid position"). All these mechanisms of defence are not typically used against the neurotic conflicts of the Oedipus complex. Instead, they are focused on avoiding a persecutory anxiety in which one's own survival is threatened.

The paranoid-schizoid position is simply a developmental phase; it is a constellation of typical relations, anxieties, and defences. It is, moreover, a position to which we may revert at specific times in our lives, for instance in wartime, bringing out a powerful sense of love directed at one's own community or nation and a quite separate, powerful hate towards an enemy.

Self

J.A.: Winnicott used the term "unit-status" to define a formed self which is distinct from the ego. The baby evolves unit-status by the stage of relative dependence, after the first three months of life. This stage of development relates to the developing capacity to distinguish Me from Not-Me. The terms Me and Not-Me were created by Winnicott as words that have an emotional meaning similar to Freud's use of "das ich" instead of "ego".

R.D.H.: Bion rarely uses the term "ego", and so, as with Klein, ego and self are for him more or less synonymous. The term "self" has a more subjective and personal connotation. Freud views the ego as the executive agent within the personality, managing the relations between id, super-ego, and reality. But for Kleinians there is a more experiential quality to the management of anxiety. Often, "ego" refers merely the personality that, for example, turns on itself to prevent one of its functions generating anxiety.

Survival-of-the-object

J.A.: At the core of Winnicott's paper "The use of an object" is the notion of "survival-of-the-object". This concept sets out an alternative concept to that of the death instinct for both Freud and Klein. The development and integration of the individual's innate, benign aggression depends on *survival-of-the-object*.

Surviving and non surviving objects

Abram, 2022, proposed the terms "surviving object" and "non surviving object" to extend Winnicott's inference in his work on the use of an object and *survival-of-the-object*. She designates the surviving object as an intrapsychic subjective object that emanates from the object's interpsychic survival of the infant's ruthless needs. Conversely, the non surviving object – also an intrapsychic subjective object – emanates from the object's non survival in the early interpsychic relationship. The specifics of the interpsychic dynamic that take place in the early parent-infant relationship constitutes the foundations of human development that will be revivified in the transference-countertransference matrix of the analytic relationship (Abram, 2013, ch. 14).

Symbolisation

R.D.H.: The colleagues of Klein who first applied the theory of schizoid mechanisms in work with psychotic states had to note the symptoms typical of the psychiatric diagnoses. For instance, the loss of reality was a particular interest of Bion's. In a parallel way, Hanna Segal took an interest in the problems of symbolic thinking. Bion agreed with this as a significant characteristic. He was therefore interested in the failure of symbolisation as it was expressed in the concrete entities he called beta-elements (see "paranoid-schizoid position").

The creation of symbols by human minds entails a function by which one thing is allowed to be "as if" it is another. A word heard as a phonetic sequence, such as "oak tree", is immediately processed by the listener by bringing to mind the image of an oak tree and all its association for them. Such a function fails in the schizophrenic condition, and words become exactly the thing they are supposed to represent. Even in ordinary conversation, when it gets heated, swear words can be used which have nothing to do with their actual religious meaning or with sexual parts and functioning. Nevertheless, such words have an impact that is quasi-physical and can cause wounds in the listener's sense of himself. In psychotic states, such words are felt to be actually physical missiles that harm and wound others. Bion adopted these characteristics for what he termed "beta-elements", which in psychotic states cannot be processed by the alpha-function because that function has been put out of action by the subject himself in order to avoid certain anxieties which might fill the mind if the function were performed.

Theoretical first feed

J.A.: This is a term Winnicott used to denote the very beginnings of symbolic thinking and symbolisation in the newborn infant. The theoretical first feed is a culmination of needs met through the mother's adaptation to need. It is associated with "creating the object" and the illusion of omnipotence.

Transitional phenomena and transitional objects

J.A.: One of Winnicott's well-known concepts that refers to an intermediate dimension of living. Transitionality refers to the infant's emotional journey from being merged with the mother to developing the capacity to distinguish Me from Not-Me. The transitional object refers to the infant's choice of an object that aids this journey (for example, the teddy bear).

Unconscious phantasy

J.A.: Winnicott did not subscribe to the proposal that unconscious phantasy was innate because his view was that the infant's experience of the m/other was at the root of imagination and illusion, and the ability to play and grow, in sharp distinction to delusion, the inability to play, and the lack of development.

R.D.H.: Bion adopted the notion of narrative phantasies as the basic constituents of the unconscious mind (in fact, probably of the mind itself). As Susan Isaacs explained in the "First paper of the Controversial Discussions" in 1943, instincts are represented as phantasies. This was a groundbreaking step in formulating the move from a distinct psychology (as classical psychoanalysis was becoming) towards an object-relations school (something the British Psychoanalytical Society had been harbouring and nourishing). This divergence was initiated by the development of the play technique by Klein for the analysis of young children. The child played out phantasies in a creative way, like dreams, to show the basis of its mental activity as an unconscious narrative – typically, the story of Oedipus.

However, Klein was influenced by Karl Abraham (her second analyst), who, despite a devoted loyalty to Freud, took the various psychodynamics Freud had described and understood them as narratives. For instance, perhaps at Abraham's suggestion, Freud in 1914 described narcissism in terms of spitting out bad things and swallowing down good things. Bion's use of his countertransference (see "countertransference") helped him to understand the powerful stories his patients felt they were concretely a part of; for instance, in one case the patient, in order to avoid seeing the analyst's presence, felt his sight had been ejected (by projective identification) from his eyes and into Bion, and when Bion spoke, the patient felt that his own attacked and projected sight had been violently returned to him.

BIBLIOGRAPHY

Abram, J. (2021) "On Winnicott's concept of trauma". *International Journal of Psychoanalysis*, 102: 778–793.

Abram, J. (2007) *The Language of Winnicott: A Dictionary of Winnicott's Use of Words*. 2nd edn. London: Routledge.

Abram, J. (2008) "Donald Woods Winnicott (1896–1971): a brief introduction", *International Journal of Psychoanalysis*, 89: 189–1217.

Abram, J. (2013) (Ed.) *Donald Winnicott Today*. London: Routledge.

Abram, J. (2014) "Le miroir inter-analytique : Son rôle dans la reconnaissance des traumas trans-générationnels désavoués" [The inter-analytic mirror: Its role in recognising disavowed trauma], Revue française de psychanalyse, 78(2): 405–416.

Abram, J. (2022) "Abram's response to the letter to editor". *International Journal of Psychoanalysis*. 103: 383–84.

Abram, J. (2022) *The Surviving Object: Psychoanalytic Clinical Essays on Psychic Survival-of-the Object*. London and New York: Routledge.

Abram, J. and Hinshelwood R.D. (2021) International Psychoanalytic Association webinar, July 2021.

Abram, J. and Hinshelwood, R.D. (2018) *The Clinical Paradigms of Melanie Klein and Donald Winnicott: Comparisons and Dialogues*. London: Routledge.

Abram, J., Joyce, A., and Thompson, N. (2018) "Winnicott's analysis of Masud Khan: revelations from the archives". Bulletin British Psychoanalytical Society, 27 October.

Aguayo, J., de Cortinas, L.P., and Regczkey, A. (2017) *Bion in Buenos Aires*. London: Karnac.

Aguayo, J. and Malin, B. (2013) *Wilfred Bion: Los Angeles Seminars and Supervision*. London: Karnac.

Bion Talamo, P. (1997) "Aftermath". In W.R. Bion, *War Memoirs 1917–1919*: 309–312. London: Karnac.

Bion, W.R. (1948a) "Experiences in Groups: II". *Human Relations*, 1: 487–496.

Bion, W.R. (1948b) "Experiences in Groups: II". *Human Relations*, 1: 487–496.

Bion, W.R. (1948c) "Group methods of treatment". In Flugel, J.C. (Ed) *Proceedings of the International Conference on Medical Psychotherapy*: 106–109. Republished in W.R. Bion (2014) *The Complete Works of W.R. Bion*. Volume IV. London: Karnac: 65–70.

Bion, W.R. (1952) "Group dynamics: a review". *International Journal of Psychoanalysis*, 33: 235–247. Revised and reprinted M. Klein, P. Heimann, and R. Money-Kyrle (eds) (1955) *New Directions in Psychoanalysis*. New York: Basic Books; and in W.R. Bion (1961) *Experiences in Groups*. London: Tavistock.

Bion, W.R. (1957) "Differentiation of the psychotic form the non-psychotic parts of the ego". *International Journal of Psychoanalysis*, 38: 266–275

Bion, W.R. (1958) "On hallucination". *International Journal of Psychoanalysis*, 39: 341–349.

Bion, W.R. (1959) "Attacks on linking". *International Journal of Psychoanalysis*, 40: 308–315.

Bion, W.R. (1961) *Experiences in Groups and Other Papers*. London: Tavistock.

Bion, W.R. (1962a) *Learning from Experience*. London: Heinemann.

Bion, W.R. (1962b) "A psychoanalytic study of thinking". *International Journal of Psychoanalysis*, 43: 306–310. Republished as "A theory of thinking" in W.R. Bion (1967) *Second Thoughts*. London: Heinemann: 110–119.

Bion, W.R. (1963) *Elements of Psycho-Analysis*. London: Heinemann.

Bion, W.R. (1965) *Transformations*. London: Tavistock.

Bion, W.R. (1967) *Second Thoughts*. London: Heinemann.

Bion, W.R. (1970) *Attention and Interpretation*. London: Tavistock.

Bion, W.R. (1975) *A Memoir of the Future, Book 1: The Dream*. Rio de Janeiro: Imago.

Bion, W.R. (1977) *A Memoir of the Future, Book 2: The Past Presented*. Rio de Janeiro: Imago.

Bion, W.R. (1979) *A Memoir of the Future, Book 3: The Dawn of Oblivion*. New York and Sao Paolo: Clunie Press.

Bion, W.R. (1982) *The Long Weekend 1897–1919*. Abingdon: Fleetwood.

Bion, W.R. (1985) *All my Sins Remembered: Another Part of a Life*. Abingdon: Fleetwood Press.

Bion, W.R. (1992) *Cogitations*. London: Karnac.

Bion, W.R. (1997) *War Memoirs*. London: Karnac.

Bion, W.R. and Rickman, J. (1943) "Intragroup tensions in groups". *Lancet ii*: 678–681.

Bollas, C. (2002) *Free association*. London: Icon.

Bollas, C. (2007) *The Freudian moment*. London: Karnac.

Brierley, M. (1937) "Affects in Theory and Practice". *International Journal of Psychoanalysis*, 18: 256–268

Brown, J.A.C. (1964) *Freud and the Post-Freudians*. London: Penguin.

Culbert-Koehn, J. (2011). "An analysis with Bion: An interview with James Gooch". *Journal of Analytic Psychology*, 56(1): 76–91.

Dicks, H.V. (1970) *Fifty Years of the Tavistock Clinic*. London: Tavistock.

Ezriel, H. (1956) "Experimentation within the psychoanalytic session". *British Journal for the Philosophy of Science*, 7: 29–48.

Faimberg, H. (1996) "Listening to listening". *International Journal of Psychoanalysis*, 77: 667–677.

Feldman, M. (2007) "Addressing parts of the self". *International Journal of Psychoanalysis*, 88: 371–386.

Ferenczi, S., Abraham, K., Simmel, E., and Jones, E. (1921). *Psychoanalysis of the War Neurosis*. London: International Psychoanalytical Press.

Freud, A. (1927) Einführung in die Technik der Kinderanalyse. Vienna: Internationaler psychoanalytischer Verlag. Published in English as A. Freud (1928) *Introduction to the Technique of Child Analysis*. New York: Nervous and Mental Disease Publishing Company, and A. Freud (1946) *The Psycho-Analytic Treatment of Children*. London: Imago.

Freud, S. (1911) "Formulations on the two principles of mental functioning". Republushed in S. Freud (1953) *The Standard Edition of the Complete Psychological Works of Sigmund Freud*. Volume XIII. London: Hogarth: 213–226.

Freud, S. (1912) "Recommendations to physicians practising psycho-analysis". Republished in S. Freud (1953) *The Standard Edition of the Complete Psychological Works of Sigmund Freud*. Volume XII. London: Hogarth: 109–120

Freud, S. (1914) "Group influences and the maladjusted child: the school aspect". *On Narcissism. The Standard Edition of the Complete Psychological Works of Sigmund Freud*. Volume 14. London: Hogarth: 67–102.

Freud, S. (1915) "The unconscious". Republished in S. Freud (1953) *The Standard Edition of the Complete Psychological Works of Sigmund Freud*. Volume XIV. London: Hogarth:159–215.

Freud, S. (1917) "Lecture 28, Analytic therapy". In S. Freud (1953) *Introductory Lectures on Psychoanalysis. The Standard Edition of the Complete Psychological Works of Sigmund Freud*. Volume XVI. London: Hogarth: 241–463.

Freud, S. (1923) "The Ego and the Id". In S. Freud (1953) *The Standard Edition of the Complete Psychological Works of Sigmund Freud.* Volume 19. London: Hogarth: 12–66.

Freud, S. (1927) "The Future of an Illusion". In S. Freud (1953) *The Standard Edition of the Complete Psychological Works of Sigmund Freud*. Volume 21. London: Hogarth: 3–56.

Freud, S. (1937) "Constructions in Analysis". *SE,* 23: 261.

Freud, S. (1938) "An Outline of Psycho-Analysis". In S. Freud (1953) The Standard Edition of the Complete Works of Sigmund Freud. Volume 23. London: Hogarth: 141–207.

Gillespie, W. (1972) "Commemorative Meeting for Dr. Donald Winnicott, January 19th 1972". *Scientific Bulletin,* 19 January.

Green, A. (1975) "Potential space in psychoanalysis: The object in the setting". In S. Grolnick and L. Barkin (Eds) *Between Reality and Fantasy*. New York: Jason Aronson: 169–189.

Green, A. (2000) "The posthumous Winnicott: On human nature". In J. Abram (Ed) *André Green at the Squiggle Foundation.* London: Karnac: 69–83.

Green, A. (2005) "Science and science fiction in infant research". In J. Sandler, A.-M. Sandler, and R. Davies (Eds) *Clinical and Observational Psychoanalytic Research Roots of a Controversy*: London: Karnac Books.

Grunbaum, A. (1984) *Foundations of Psychoanalysis.* Berkeley and Los Angeles: California University Press.

Harris Williams, M. (2010) *Bion's Dream A Reading of the Autobiographies.* London: Karnac.

Heimann, P. (1950) "On counter-transference". *International Journal of Psychoanalysis*, 31: 81–84.

Hinshelwood, R.D. (1989) *A Dictionary of Kleinian Thought*. London: Free Association Books.

Hinshelwood, R.D. (2013) *Research on the Couch.* London: Routedge.

Hinshelwood, R.D. (2018) "John Rickman behind the scenes: The influence of Lewin's field theory on practice, countertransference and W.R. Bion". *International Journal of Psychoanalysis*, 100: 1409–1423.

Hinshelwood, R.D. (2022) *W.R. Bion as Clinician: Steering between Concepts and Practice.* London: Routledge.

Jones, E. (1935) "Early female sexuality". *International Journal of Psychoanalysis,* 16: 263–273.

Joseph, B. (1978) "Different types of anxiety and their handling in the analytic situation". *International Journal of PsychoAnalysis*, 59: 2223–2228.

Joseph, B. (1989) *Psychic Equilibrium and Psychic Change*. London: Routledge.

Jung, C.G. (1968) *Analytical Psychology: Its Theory and Practice.* New York: Pantheon.

Kahr, B. (1996). *DW Winnicott: A Biographical Portrait*. London: Karnac.

King, P. (1972) "Tribute to Donald Winnicott Commemorative Meeting". *Scientific Bulletin*, 19 January.

Klein, M. (1929) "Personification in the Play of Children". *International Journal of Psychoanalysis*, 10: 193–204.

Klein, M. (1932) *The Psychoanalysis of Children*. London: Hogarth.

Klein, M. (1935) "A contribution to the genesis of manic-depressive states". *The International Journal of Psychoanalysis*, 16: 145–174.

Klein, M. (1946) "Notes on some schizoid mechanisms". *International Journal of Psychoanalysis*, 27: 99–110.

Malin, B. (2021) R. B. Braithwaite's influence on Bion's epistemological contributions. *Int Jl of Psychoanal* 102: 653–670.

Milner, M. (1972) "Commemorative Meeting for Dr. Donald Winnicott". *Scientific Bulletin*, 19 January.

Ogden, T.H. (2001) "Reading Winnicott". *Psychoanalytc Quarterly*, 70: 299–323.

Ogden, T.H. (2022) *Coming to Life in the Consulting Room: Toward a New Analytic Sensibility*. London: Routledge.

Perelberg, R. (2015) *Murdered Father, Dead Father Revisiting the Oedipus Complex*. London: Routledge.

Popper, K. (1959) *The Logic of Scientific Discovery*. London: Hutchinson.

Rodman, F.R. (Ed) (1987) *The Spontaneous Gesture: Selected letters of DW Winnicott*. Cambridge: Harvard University Press.

Rodman, R. (2003) *Winnicott: Life and Work*. Cambridge: Perseus Publishing.

Segal, H. (1978) "On symbolism". *International Journal of Psychoanalysis*, 59: 315–319.

Segal, H. (1983) "Some clinical implications of Melanie Klein's work – Emergence from narcissism". *International Journal of Psychoanalysis*, 64: 269–276.

Steiner, J. (1993) *Psychic Retreats*. London: Routledge.

Steiner, J. (2000) "Containment, enactment and communication". *International Journal of Psychoanal*ysis, 81: 245–255.

Steiner, J. (2017) *Lectures on Technique by Melanie Klein*. London: Routledge.

Strachey, J. (1934) "The nature of the therapeutic action of psychoanalysis". *International Journal of Psychoanal*, 15: 127–159.

Strachey, J. (1975) "Appendix C: Words and things". In S, Freud (1953) *The Standard Edition of the Complete Psychological Works of Sigmund Freud*. Volume XIV. London: Hogarth: 209–215.

Tustin, F. (1981) "A modern pilgrim's progress: Reminiscences of personal analysis with Dr. Bion". *Journal of Child Psychotherapy*, 7: 175–179.

Vonofakos, D. and. Hinshelwood, R.D. (2012) "Wilfred Bion's letters to John Rickman (1939–1951)". *Psychoanalysis and History*, 14: 53–94.

Wilden, A. (1973) *System and Structure: Essays in Communication and Exchange*. London: Tavistock.

Winnicott, C. (1978) "D.W.W.: A reflection". In S.A. Grolnink and L. Barkin (Eds) *Between Reality and Fantasy: Transitional Objects and Phenomena*. New York: Aronson: 17–33.

Winnicott, C., Shepherd, R., and Davis, M. (1989) *Psychoanalytic Explorations*. Cambridge: Harvard University Press.

Winnicott, D.W. (1941) "The observation of infants in a set situation". International Journal of Psychoanalysis, 22: 229–249.

Winnicott, D.W. (1945) "Primitive emotional development". *International Journal of Psychoanalysis*, 26: 137–143.

Winnicott, D.W. (1946) "Letter to Ella Sharpe". In F.R. Rodman (Ed) (1978) *The Spontaneous Gesture: Selected Letters*. Cambridge: Harvard University Press.

Winnicott, D.W. (1949a) "Birth Memories, Birth Trauma, and Anxiety". In D.W. Winnicott (1958) *Collected Papers: Through Paediatrics to Psychoanalysis*. London: Tavistock: 174–193.

Winnicott, D.W. (1952) "Psychoses and child care". *British Journal of Medical Psychology*, 26: 68–74.

Winnicott, D.W. (1955) "Group influences and the maladjusted child". In *The Family and Individual Development*. London: Tavistock, 146–154.

Winnicott, D.W. (1956) "Primary maternal preoccupation". In C. Winnicott, R. Shepherd, and M. Davis (Eds) *Psychoanalytic Explorations*. Cambridge: Harvard University Press: 300–305.

Winnicott, D.W. (1957) *The Child and the Outside World: Studies in Developing Relationships*. London: Tavistock.

Winnicott, D.W. (1958) *Collected Papers: Through Paediatrics to Psychoanalysis*. London: Tavistock.

Winnicott, D.W. (1960) "The theory of the parent-infant relationship". *International Journal Psychoanalysis*, 41: 585–595.

Winnicott, D.W. (1965a) *The Maturational Processes and The Facilitating Environment: Studies in the Theory of Emotional Development*. London: Hogarth.

Winnicott, D.W. (1965b) "A personal view of the Kleinian contribution". In *The Maturational Processes and The Facilitating Environment: Studies in the Theory of Emotional Development*: London: Hogarth: 171–178.

Winnicott, D.W. (1966) "The ordinary devoted mother". In C. Winnicott, R. Shepherd and, M. Davis (Eds) (1987) *Psychoanalytic Explorations*. Cambridge: Harvard University Press: 51–58.

Winnicott, D.W. (1969a) "The use of an object". *International Journal of Psychoanalysis*, 50: 711–716.

Winnicott, D.W. (1969b) "Obituary: James Strachey". International Journal of Psychoanalysis, 50: 508.

Winnicott, D.W. (1970) "Cure". In D.W. Winnicott, *Collected Works of Donald Winnicott*. Volume 9. Oxford: Oxford University Press: 2–10.

Winnicott, D.W. (1971a) *Playing and Reality*. London: Tavistock.

Winnicott, D.W. (1971b) "Basis for self in body". In D.W. Winnicott, *Collected Works of Donald Winnicott*. Volume 9. Oxford: Oxford University Press: 225–234.

Winnicott, D.W. (1971c) *Therapeutic Consultations in Child Psychiatry*. London: Hogarth.

Winnicott, D.W. (1986) "Home is where we start from". In C, Winnicott, R. Shepherd and, M. Davis (Eds) *Essays by a Psychoanalyst*. Reading: Addison-Wesley: 259–261.

Winnicott, D.W. (1987) "Babies and their mothers". In C. Winnicott, R. Shepherd, and M. Davis (Eds.) *Psychoanalytic Explorations*. Cambridge: Harvard University Press: 96–102.

Winnicott, D.W. (1989) "Postscript: DWW on DWW". In C. Winnicott, R. Shepherd and M. Davis (Eds.) *Psychoanalytic Explorations*. Cambridge: Harvard University Press: 569–582.

Winnicott, D.W. and Britton C (1947) "Residential management as treatment for difficult children". In D.W. Winnicott (1965a) *The Maturational Processes and The Facilitating Environment: Studies in the Theory of Emotional Development*. London: Hogarth: 77–94.

INDEX

Note: Page numbers in **bold** indicate tables on the corresponding pages

For Product Safety Concerns and Information please contact our EU
representative GPSR@taylorandfrancis.com
Taylor & Francis Verlag GmbH, Kaufingerstraße 24, 80331 München, Germany

www.ingramcontent.com/pod-product-compliance
Ingram Content Group UK Ltd.
Pitfield, Milton Keynes, MK11 3LW, UK
UKHW020139200926
475702UK00005B/822

* 9 7 8 1 0 3 2 4 6 5 8 0 7 *